The DASH Diet to End Obesity

Advance Praise for *The DASH Diet to End Obesity*

"Twenty years ago Dr. William M. Manger was studying and battling the hypertension plague in America when he discovered that a tsunami of blubber was heading our way. He sounded the alarm. Not enough people listened, and the tsunami, code named Obesity, hit with full catastrophic force. But now Dr. Manger and his three distinguished colleagues have found a way out for citizens drowning in the lipid ooze—and Dr. Manger is an exemplar of his own advice. After ninety-two years his dermis still fits him like a surfer's wetsuit. He has a surfer's muscles, too. Pound for pound, age-adjusted, he is the strongest man east of the Alleghenies."

— Thomas K. Wolfe, Jr., Author
New York, NY

"This is an outstanding book, both for its content and for ease of reading. Everyone can make use of the information and recommendations it contains. The book provides guidance for all of us who want to take responsibility for our behaviors and eating habits. The result will be better health. Additionally, the book makes a strong case for the importance of instituting nationwide efforts in one or more of the following areas: to reduce sodium in all foods, to increase exercise in schools, and to emphasize nutrition education in schools. These efforts, viewed as investments in our future, will pay dividends in healthier citizens and a more competitive workforce."

— Denis A. Cortese, MD
Foundation Professor and Director of Arizona State University
Healthcare Delivery and Policy Program
President of the Healthcare Transformation Institute
Emeritus President and CEO Mayo Clinic
Rochester, MN

"The American diet includes too much salt and too-large portions. Obesity is a new American public health problem, increasing one's risk of heart disease and cancer. This book on the commonsense DASH diet (with great tables and pictures) can help you adopt a healthy diet to mitigate your risk of hypertension, cardiovascular disease, and cancer—and to make you feel (and look) better!"

— Karen H. Antman, MD
Provost, Medical Campus
Dean, School of Medicine
Boston University School of Medicine
Boston, MA

"This is a book that every family should read and every institution, both public and private, should own. The authors have been at the forefront of trying to solve the problem of obesity. It seems to me that some people and some industries are finally starting to wake up to this problem and the effect it has on the individual and on society. This book is easy and clear to read, and full of facts that should propel us all into action."

— Sissel Cooper Bos
Director of the Irving S. Cooper Family Foundation
Naples, FL

"This book is an extraordinary collection of what to do for obesity from the standpoint of the patient, the managing physician, and the caregiver. The information ranges from the complications of obesity to what exactly to do about it—and what not to do. It evaluates many popular diets. Just in case you can't remember which fats are the good kind and which are undesirable, this book has the answers. And, finally, the politics of obesity are discussed as an area of potential improvement."

— John W. Braasch, MD, PhD
Former Chief of Surgery, Lahey Clinic

"For half a century I have been familiar with the wide scope of Dr. William Manger's intelligence, his analytical prowess, and his deep medical knowledge. He is motivated principally by curiosity and compassion. It is important for us all that Bill Manger and his associates have applied laserlike attention to the scourge of obesity with his new book, *The DASH Diet to End Obesity*. It opened my eyes—wide."

— Walter J.P. Curley
U.S. Ambassador to Ireland (1975–77)
And to France (1989–93)

"This book is wonderful. The style and quality seem right on target."

— Lewis R. Goldfrank, MD
Chairman, Department of Emergency Medicine, NYU School of Medicine
Director, Department of Emergency Medicine,
Bellevue Hospital
New York, NY

"If we are to solve the health-care crisis, the key is to make all of us healthier. Preventive medicine should be our first priority, encompassing proper diet, exercise, avoidance of smoking, and moderating intake of alcohol and drugs. This book clearly and thoroughly tells us how to accomplish these goals. It is written in terms understandable by the public, but is also a useful guide for health-care professionals. It should be used as a text in grade-school health programs, as habits developed in children are likely to persist for life."

— Robert S. Gordon, MD
Late Associate Clinical Professor of Medicine
Yale School of Medicine

"*The DASH Diet to End Obesity* is the good nutrition bible."

— Catherine and Oliver Grant
Mr. Grant is former Director of Athletics at St. Albans School
Washington, D.C.

"Thank you for writing *The DASH Diet to End Obesity*. It is an important fusion of common sense, biology, and public health, and a major contribution to the national dialogue on what it means to be a healthy society."

— Henry S. Lodge, MD
Associate Clinical Professor Specializing in Internal Medicine and Prevention
Columbia University College of Physicians and Surgeons
New York, NY

"The book is clearly written, offers a number of sensible approaches to a major health problem, and contains many practical tips that can prove useful. If it has a beneficial effect on even a small percentage of its readers, the authors will be able to take satisfaction in knowing that they have accomplished something."

— John N. Loeb, MD
Emeritus Professor of Medicine
Columbia University College of Physicians & Surgeons
New York, NY

"The authors have produced a superb and in-depth text that defines the magnitude and rapid increase of obesity and its myriad complications in America and elsewhere. The book describes in detail the DASH eating plan, which, in association with physical activity and other lifestyle changes, shows great promise as part of a comprehensive approach to ameliorating the burgeoning problem of obesity. The section describing many popular but flawed alternative diets is also highly informative. The book correctly points to the crucial role of early intervention and personal responsibility. This is a timely and important book given the enormous and growing scale of obesity-related health problems in the U.S., which threaten not just our physical well-being but also our nation's economy."

— Jules Manger, MD
Retired emergency physician
Past director emergency department and co-director trauma service
Concord Hospital, Concord, NH
Founding partner and past president Concord Emergency Medical Associates
Past director emergency medical services for central NH
Former adjunct teaching staff Dartmouth Medical School

"This book is well written, easy to understand, and proof that our health's destiny is ours to control."

— Matthew Fraher Minno, Esq.
Deputy General Counsel
Florida Department of Management Services
Tallahassee, FL

"We know from carefully controlled research that the DASH diet offers important benefits for blood pressure and weight loss. But the real challenge people face in trying to change their eating habits is sticking with it. This book provides, in simple language and through practical hints, the information and motivation that people need to follow the DASH diet in their daily lives. It is a major contribution."

— Thomas J. Moore, MD
Associate Provost, Boston University Medical Center
Chairman of the DASH Trial and Founder of DASHforHealth.com
tmoore@bu.edu

"*The DASH Diet to End Obesity* sets forth in straight talk ways to prevent the horrors of the obesity epidemic and its often deadly complications. The book also touches on how to deal with the psychiatric and emotional implications of obesity, such as low self-esteem, depression, social isolation, peer criticism, and rejection—all of which can make life miserable for people of all ages. Information about the importance of preventing obesity at a young age and combating it later in life offer the readers of this book hope and a way out."

— The late Berthold E. Schwarz, AB, MD, MS
Former Psychiatrist
Vero Beach, FL

The DASH Diet Eating Plan is Recommended by
American Heart Association • National Cancer Institute
National Institutes of Health • National Hypertension Association
United States Department of Agriculture
Leading medical centers • Registered dieticians

DEDICATION

*To my grandchildren—Samantha, Catherine, and Jackson—
and for all those children and adults who opt to improve
their lifestyles and strengthen the health of our nation.*

*And to my wife, Lynn, for her remarkable expertise
in skillfully developing the curriculum for the VITAL
(Values Initiative Teaching About Lifestyle)
program to improve the lifestyles of young children by teaching
them healthy eating and appropriate physical activity—
an extremely important and very noble cause.*

BILL MANGER

The DASH* Diet *to* End Obesity

THE <u>BEST</u> PLAN TO PREVENT HYPERTENSION AND TYPE 2 DIABETES AND REDUCE EXCESS WEIGHT

WILLIAM M. MANGER, MD, PHD
JENNIFER K. NELSON, MS, RD
MARION J. FRANZ, MS, RD, CDE
EDWARD J. ROCCELLA, PHD, MPH

Hunter House
PUBLISHERS

*Dietary Approaches to Stop Hypertension

Hunter House Inc., Publishers
PO Box 2914
Alameda CA 94501-0914

Library of Congress Cataloging-in-Publication Data
The DASH diet to end obesity : the best plan to prevent hypertension and type 2
diabetes and reduce excess weight / William M. Manger [and three others].
pages cm
"Recommended by: American Heart Association, National Cancer Institute, National
Institutes of Health, National Hypertension Association, U.S. Department of
Agriculture, leading medical centers, and registered dietitians."
Includes index.
ISBN 978-0-89793-643-9 (pbk.) — ISBN 978-0-89793-693-4 (ebook)
1. Reducing diets. 2. Hypertension—Diet therapy. 3. Diabetes—Diet therapy.
I. Manger, William Muir, 1920-
RM222.2.D2987 2013
616.4'620654—dc23   2013029726

Project Credits

Cover Design: Brian Dittmar Design	Acquisitions Intern: Sally Castillo
Book Production: John McKercher	Rights Coordinator: Candace Groskreutz
Developmental Reviewers: Mary Claire	Publisher's Assistant: Bronwyn Emery
Blakeman, Jude Berman	Publicity Coordinator: Martha Scarpati
Developmental and Copy Editor:	Customer Service Manager:
Kelley Blewster	Christina Sverdrup
Indexer: Candace Hyatt	Order Fulfillment: Washul Lakdhon
Managing Editor: Alexandra Mummery	Administrator: Theresa Nelson
Editorial Intern: Jordan Collins	IT Support: Peter Eichelberger
Publisher: Kiran S. Rana	

Printed and bound by Sheridan Books, Ann Arbor, Michigan
Manufactured in the United States of America

9 8 7 6 5 4 3 2 1   First Edition   14 15 16 17 18

▶ Contents

▶ Foreword *by Dr. John N. Schullinger*

If you would take the time to read this book, it could add many healthy years to your life and might even pull you back from the brink of losing it. Within these pages you will find a reader-friendly, up-to-date compilation of knowledge and advice on conditions that threaten our lives and ways to avoid them. You will learn about the "deadly quartet" (obesity, diabetes, elevated blood fats, and high blood pressure) and the importance of seeking prompt medical treatment and adopting a healthier lifestyle. This is *not* a book about a new diet or weight-loss medication. Rather, it is a guide to a full and healthy life through good nutrition, attainable levels of exercise, and the avoidance of controllable risk factors, which can only lead to premature disability and death.

Most important, this book is an exhortation to take responsibility for our own health and the health of our children. The consequences of not doing so can be devastating.

This book, I believe, should be in every school library and, if possible, in every home. Dr. Manger and his team of experts have presented for us in this one volume the information we need to understand why and how we may lead long, productive, and healthy lives. We should take this information to "heart."

— John N. Schullinger, MD, FACP, FACC
Emeritus Professor of Pediatrics
Columbia Presbyterian Medical Center, New York, NY

▶ Foreword *by Dr. James R. Sowers*

Approximately two-thirds of adult Americans are overweight or obese. This state of malnutrition contributes substantially to the high prevalence of chronic disease conditions such as type 2 diabetes mellitus, hypertension, heart disease, stroke, chronic kidney disease, cancer, neurodegenerative disease, and osteoarthritis. Therefore, it is imperative to develop national health strategies to lessen overweight and obesity in the United States and the rest of the world.

This compilation of the health benefits of a DASH diet and exercise strategy offers such a potential national health initiative. We know from randomized controlled clinical research that the DASH diet offers important benefits for reducing blood pressure and aiding weight loss. In lay language, this book provides a straightforward strategy—a practical and utilitarian approach to optimal weight management, in concert with other aspects of a healthy lifestyle. It provides empowering information and motivation that will help people to follow the DASH diet in their daily lives. Dr. Manger and his three distinguished colleagues have crafted a readable approach to a healthy lifestyle which I strongly endorse.

This book should be a part of hospital, medical, and nursing teaching centers and public-health libraries throughout the nation.

— James R. Sowers, MD, FACP
Professor of Medicine, Physiology and Pharmacology
Director of the Diabetes and Cardiovascular Center
University of Missouri School of Medicine, Columbia, MO

► Acknowledgments

Jennifer Nelson, MS, RD, LD, one of the leading dietitians in the country, serves in the Department of Nutrition at the Mayo Clinic in Rochester, Minnesota. Her knowledge of nutrition is unmatched, and her consultation and guidance have been invaluable.

Marion Franz, MS, RD, LD, CDE, is also one of the nation's foremost nutritionists. She chairs Nutrition Concepts by Franz, Inc., in Minneapolis, Minnesota, and she is a leading authority on nutritional therapy for the prevention and management of diabetes mellitus.

Edward J. Roccella, PhD, MPH, deserves enormous thanks for a very detailed and constructive review of the text and statements in this book. Having formerly served at the National Institutes of Health as Coordinator of the National High Blood Pressure Education Program for many years, and having published extensively on topics dealing with hypertension, he is eminently qualified to critically proofread and contribute to the contents of this book.

Siri Sirichanvimol, MS, RD, former Clinical Manager of Nutrition at New York University Medical Center, in New York City, also contributed significantly to the nutrition guidelines in this book.

Additionally, we wish to express our deep gratitude to Thomas Moore, MD, Professor of Medicine at Boston University School of Medicine and one of the developers of the DASH diet, for his contribution to this book and his very helpful comments on healthy nutrition and dietary management.

We wish to thank Terry Seltzer, MD, Professor of Medicine and diabetes specialist, and Michael Schloss, MD, Clinical Professor of Medicine and specialist in lipid (cholesterol and triglyceride) metabolism, both at New York University Medical Center, for their consultation and advice.

We are most grateful to Richard Ruge, a distinguished lawyer and a former managing editor of *The Harvard Crimson,* and Paul Piazza, St. Albans School Associate Headmaster Emeritus and former Chairman of the English Department, for kindly proofreading this manuscript for grammatical structure. Very special thanks to my office administrator and secretary, Alla Krayko, for her skillful help in preparing the manuscript of this book. Thanks also to Robert Turecamo, Assistant Director of Development of the National Hypertension Association, for proofreading the manuscript.

We are profoundly grateful to Lynn Manger for her remarkable expertise in developing and implementing the VITAL (Values Initiative Teaching About Lifestyle) program to prevent and combat obesity in young children. Her contribution is largely responsible for the great success of VITAL.

Also, we wish to express our deep gratitude to Kelley Blewster for her extraordinarily helpful guidance in editing and improving the presentation of many parts of this book and to the other very important staff of Hunter House, whose wise suggestions are very much appreciated.

Also, we are deeply grateful for the extraordinarily helpful participation and guidance of Oliver (Skip) Grant in skillfully promoting and introducing the VITAL program to young schoolchildren. As the former Director of Athletics at St. Albans School, in Washington, D.C., he established a standard of athletic excellence and moral character in all the boys he coached so well and with such concern for good. His example as a coach and mentor was unmatched. We are reminded of a fitting quotation by the great humanitarian Albert Schweitzer: "Example is not the main thing in influencing others, it is the *only* thing."

— William M. Manger, MD, PhD, FACP, FACC

▶ Introduction

*May you and all of us be enabled to lead
our young people along a better, more noble path.*
— The Late Canon Charles Martin
    Revered and beloved Headmaster of St. Albans School

▶ Our nation was built primarily on "family, faith, and hard work"; furthermore, the remarkable success of this democracy depends, to a very large extent, on the freedom we all enjoy so much. People in all parts of the world desire and seek freedom as central to happiness. However, most would agree that freedom without responsibility is unworkable and can eventually lead only to decadence and the deterioration of any society. My late brother, Jules Manger, used to say that to complement the Statue of Liberty on the East Coast of the United States we should also have a Statue of Responsibility on the West Coast. In my opinion, his suggestion was right on target because we all should appreciate, more than ever, the crucial role of responsibility in our lives and the lives of our children.

Within the past few decades, there are increasing signs that responsibility, in a variety of areas, is not a major concern of many Americans. Erosion of belief in values and responsibility can undermine and sap the strength of our nation. We face a very serious health crisis involving diseases that often result from detrimental lifestyles. Caring for these diseases has created an enormous financial burden on the public and on our government. It is essential that we all work together to stem this medical crisis, which continues to increase.

The importance of healthy lifestyles to preserve the well-being of Americans has never been more evident. Today the United States is one of the fattest nations in the world: 68 percent of Americans are overweight and 34 percent are obese (that is, at least 20 percent above ideal weight). Complications of the obesity crisis (hypertension, type 2 diabetes, harmful blood fats, and many cancers) kill three hundred thousand Americans each year and cost the nation $190 billion. It is estimated that of children born in our nation in the year 2000, about one-third of Caucasians and one-half of African Americans and Hispanics will develop type 2 diabetes if excess weight gain continues. It is possible that parents will live longer lives than their children!

The purpose of this book is to encourage, educate, and empower American adults and children to seek healthier lifestyles, which can play a pivotal role in reducing the prevalence and complications of obesity. A top priority is to prevent childhood obesity. Chapters 1 through 3 take an in-depth look at the *problem:* the nationwide (soon-to-be worldwide) crisis of obesity, with all of its attendant health problems. Chapters 4 and 5 introduce and examine the *solution:* the best eating plan for combating obesity, which we have concluded is the DASH (Dietary Approaches to Stop Hypertension) diet. Chapters 6 through 9 cover significant related topics: other weight-loss plans, the importance of exercise, DASH for diabetes, and the salt story. In the very few instances where the singular pronoun "I" is used, it refers to me, William Manger.

This book addresses the very core of our well-being—namely, our lifestyle. The basic and vital information and recommendations outlined here provide important guidance for those interested in improving their health and that of their family. Success by adherence to a healthy lifestyle depends on persistent motivation, which, of course, is up to you. However, it must be appreciated that a low income, unhealthy eating habits (inside or outside the home), and limited access to healthy foods may make adhering to a healthy eating program very difficult for some. Addressing those important sociological issues, which have been competently written about elsewhere, is beyond the scope of this book.

This book is written, with the help of many outstanding consultants with a wide range of expertise, to improve the health of our nation by establishing beneficial lifestyles. Francis Bacon said, "Some books are to be tasted, others to be swallowed, and some few to be chewed and digested." I pray that this book is worthy of the latter category.

1 ▶ **Your** Life, Your Choices

▶ You can improve your health! This truth should be clear to all Americans. You and only you can change your lifestyle, your way of life. Regrettably, in some parts of the world many die from lack of food and malnutrition, and from various diseases because of inadequate prevention and lack of medicines, immunizations, vitamins, and sanitation. Fortunately, most Americans do not face these issues. In contrast, Americans today often die from the consequences of obesity caused by too much food, fat, and sugar, or from excess alcohol, excess salt, and lack of physical activity. They also succumb to cigarette smoking, illicit drugs, some sexually transmitted infections, and preventable injuries and diseases. To repeat: *You* alone are responsible for *your* lifestyle.

Changing What You Can

You cannot change your genes, age, sex, race, or family background, but look at what you can change. You can avoid overeating; you can consume healthy foods with less saturated fat and added sugar; you can get adequate exercise; you can limit the amount of salt you eat;

you can avoid drinking alcohol excessively; you can avoid smoking cigarettes; you can avoid using marijuana or other illicit drugs; you can get adequate sleep; you can avoid acquiring sexually transmitted infections; and you can observe safety precautions to help prevent injury and disease. (Injuries are the leading cause of death in individuals under age thirty-five.) You *can*, therefore, change your lifestyle so that you will:

- live safer
- live longer
- look better
- play better
- improve your self-esteem
- increase your energy
- reduce stress

- live healthier
- feel better
- work better
- sleep better
- improve your quality of life
- enjoy better sex
- be happier

There is no doubt that your lifestyle has an enormous impact on your health. The major modifiable risk factors (obesity, sedentary lifestyle, excess consumption of salt and alcohol, cigarette smoking, illicit drugs, and risky sexual activity) increase the chance for disease. No matter what your age, it is always essential to concentrate on changing an unhealthy lifestyle to a healthy one that will improve your future health, self-esteem, and quality of life, and will benefit your family and associates.

Overeating—especially excessive consumption of fat, sweets, snacks, and sugar—and drinking lots of sugar-laden sodas, other sweetened drinks, or excess amounts of alcohol are major causes of the increase of obesity in the United States. We are correctly warned that our children are growing up in a toxic food-and-beverage environment. Sadly, "inadequate or unskilled parental supervision can leave children vulnerable to these obesigenic environmental influences."[1] We are constantly bombarded by advertisements for food, snacks, and drinks that encourage us to eat and drink more.

The abundance of inexpensive food and non-nutritious beverages, the replacement of exercise time with screen time (TV, computers, hand-held games, and cell phones), and the availability of convenient transportation create an environment that only contributes to the crisis of obesity in our nation. The result is an increase in body fat because we consume more calories than we burn.

Some experts define overeating as an eating disorder, and others do not. Prolonged daily consumption of even a modest increase in calories—which would be difficult to categorize as an eating disorder—can account for very significant weight gain in children and adults. In addition to the ill effects of overeating, there are other types of serious but relatively rare eating disorders such as anorexia nervosa (avoidance of eating, which can cause severe malnutrition and sometimes death) and bulimia (binge eating followed by discharging the food through self-induced vomiting or the excessive use of laxatives). About 90 percent of these conditions occur in white girls and young white women and are associated with extreme psychological disturbances. Anyone with either of these conditions is very fearful of gaining weight and becoming obese. In this book, we will focus only on obesity, one of our greatest health threats. To avoid obesity and maintain a normal weight, "healthy eating" rather than "dieting" should be emphasized, since dieting is occasionally the gateway to bulimia or anorexia.

Overeating in general is a serious problem, but so is overindulging in certain items. For example, excessive salt consumption can elevate blood pressure in many people, and it can aggravate or cause hypertension in individuals who are sensitive to salt. It has also been linked to gastric cancer and asthma. A high-fat diet has been linked to some cancers—especially colon cancer. Excessive alcohol consumption adds more calories and increases weight with no nutritional benefit. It also can cause or contribute to hypertension, and chronic alcoholism can damage the liver, brain, heart, and nerves.

A healthy eating plan combats *both* overeating in general *and* the overconsumption of harmful substances such as those listed above. It maintains a reasonably normal weight, which is vital to preventing or minimizing some of the most common serious diseases in Americans (more on that weighty topic in the next two chapters). It is simple to follow. There is very convincing evidence that the DASH (Dietary Approaches to Stop Hypertension) eating plan is admirably designed to meet all of these criteria. And besides helping its adherents lose weight or maintain a healthy weight, DASH can reduce elevated blood pressure (as its name implies), improve type 2 diabetes, lower or normalize abnormal blood cholesterol and triglycerides, lessen the chance of stroke, and even minimize the risk of developing a variety of cancers. Most health experts agree that this remarkably beneficial eating plan is ideal for almost everyone. Details on the DASH eating plan are provided in Chapter 4.

Prevention Starts Early

Effective prevention is always far better than treating a disease. It is especially important for schools to provide the proper guidance and opportunity for good nutrition and exercise at a very young age—to children in preschool, kindergarten, and first and second grades, when they are particularly receptive and eager to learn, (and then reinforcing, expanding, and promoting a healthy lifestyle in all grades through high school). Early efforts to establish a healthy lifestyle in young children will reduce the chance of obesity, which is often associated with psychosocial factors (e.g., weight-related teasing, fewer friends, and depression) that degrade quality of life. Furthermore, it is reported that an obese teenager has a greater than 70 percent risk of becoming an obese adult. Another report indicates that only 15 percent of children with normal weight become obese adults, whereas 82 percent of obese children become obese adults. These facts underscore the importance of maintaining a normal weight in childhood.

Solid evidence exists showing that the obesity epidemic is affecting our nation's young people. In one recent study of American Indian children, obesity, hypertension, and abnormal elevation in blood sugar after eating were strongly linked to increased premature death (i.e., before age fifty-five).[2] One recent national survey found that more than 20 percent of adolescents twelve to nineteen years old had abnormal blood fat levels; the percent increased to 43 percent among those who were also obese.[3] Other studies indicate that obese children as young as three years old have evidence of an inflammatory response that has been linked to heart disease in later life. A troubling report found obesity in 27 percent of preschool children in New York City whose families live below the poverty line; this was especially evident in Hispanic and African American children.[4]

The importance of healthy eating and adequate exercise should be repeated and reinforced as a child grows older. At appropriate ages, education about the risks of cigarette smoking, the use of illicit drugs and alcohol, risky sexual activities, and ways of minimizing injuries should be introduced and discussed repeatedly at all subsequent grade levels until high-school graduation. Parents should make a strong effort to intervene and influence their children about healthy eating from the beginning—long before children enter school. It is important not to overfeed—crying does not necessarily indicate that a child is hungry. Parents have an obligation to participate in this vital educational process. The future lives of many children will benefit greatly by early education and implementation of healthy lifestyles. Establishing a healthy lifestyle early affords the greatest opportunity for good health throughout one's life and into future generations.

· · · · · · · · ·

Now for some good news. The National Hypertension Association has developed the VITAL program (Values Initiative Teaching About Lifestyle), which has been introduced to about thirty-five thousand young children in twelve states and the District of Columbia. The program teaches healthy eating based largely on the DASH eating plan and also emphasizes appropriate physical activity. The enthusiasm for this program shown by children, school nurses, teachers, educational professionals, pediatricians, and parents has been extremely positive and gratifying. The American Heart Association has adopted the VITAL program as part of their program to reduce childhood obesity. Preliminary results indicate that the program has had a beneficial effect on the lifestyles of young children and is very helpful in preventing overweight and obesity. (We are pleased to report that in October 2009 we received the Mayo Clinic Alumni Association Humanitarian Award for our efforts to prevent overweight and obesity in children and future generations.)

In 2000 two small towns in France started a community-based effort to prevent overweight in children by encouraging healthy eating and increased physical activity. The effort involved not only schoolteachers but almost the entire community. The result was remarkably positive: By 2005 the prevalence of overweight in children was only 8.8 percent, whereas in neighboring towns and throughout the nation it was 17.8 percent.

It is evident that efforts to prevent unhealthy lifestyles are crucial to improving the health of children and future generations. Equally important to note, however, is that these efforts can work.

. . . .

The purpose of this book is to present facts that will encourage you to take the necessary steps to change and improve your lifestyle and benefit your health and that of your family. Knowledge is power, as the saying goes. Besides learning the facts, however, know that *motivation* (a strong desire) and *persistence* (willingness to stay with it) are absolutely essential for success in achieving and maintaining a healthy lifestyle. All worthwhile endeavors require effort. Remember, "Nothing works like work." Informing and educating yourself and others about the hazards of an unhealthy lifestyle and urging people to change and improve their lifestyle and health may be helpful, but, again, motivation and persistence are the keys to success, and they depend on you! If you accept these truths, you can achieve better health and greater happiness for yourself and your family.

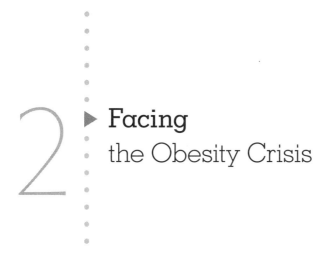

2 ▶ Facing
the Obesity Crisis

▶ Anyone reading this book has almost certainly been exposed many times to lists of the myriad problems—both individual and societal—caused by obesity. You can probably even recite most or all of these problems. Perhaps you've experienced some of them yourself firsthand. Still, as part of our goal to impart knowledge to our readers, we believe it's worthwhile for us to remind you of them once again. Maybe you're ready in a way that you weren't before to be motivated by this information to make important lifestyle changes.

Overweight and obesity are the most common nutritional problems in both underdeveloped and developed nations. In the United States, overweight (a higher-than-ideal body weight) and obesity (a body weight of at least 20 percent above the ideal) are rampant conditions. Currently there are about sixty million obese adult Americans. This is a serious health crisis. Overweight and obesity can cause or worsen the following conditions:

- hypertension (high blood pressure)
- type 2 diabetes (previously called adult-onset diabetes)
- osteoarthritis

- impaired breathing when sleeping (sometimes advancing to sleep apnea, or the periodic cessation of breathing during sleep)
- harmful changes in blood fats (cholesterol and triglycerides)
- many cancers

In turn, these conditions can trigger or worsen other health problems:

- Hypertension, diabetes, and elevated harmful blood fats result in hardening of the arteries, which can impair the blood supply to various parts of the body and lead to heart and kidney damage and failure, stroke, and poor circulation in the legs.
- Complications of arterial disease, especially damage of the arteries to the heart, brain, and kidneys, account for 50 percent of all deaths in the United States each year.
- Cancer causes about 22 percent of deaths.

More on these obesity-related health problems is provided later in the chapter.

It is alarming that, worldwide, of persons fifteen years and older, 1.6 billion are overweight and 400 million are obese; by 2015, it is predicted that 2.3 billion adults will be overweight and 700 million will be obese.

As touched on in the last chapter, some of the health risks associated with obesity are now being detected even in children, in greater numbers than ever before. In addition to the importance of early detection of hypertension and diabetes, it is recommended that every child be tested for elevated cholesterol at age ten. It is evident that overweight and obesity in children can impair self-esteem, performance in school, athletic ability, and quality of life, and it can cause peer rejection, social isolation, despair, and depression.

In the United States these complications are responsible for over three hundred thousand deaths each year—deaths for which our behavior is responsible. The annual cost of diseases attributable to obesity was reported in 2008 to be $147 billion—that is, 10 percent of the total U.S. annual medical expenses.[1] Today, the cost may be $190 billion.[2] The IRS has designated obesity as a serious disease and now allows the cost of certain weight-loss programs as a medical expense eligible for a tax deduction. As aptly stated in a recent editorial: "Fat is a fiscal issue."[3]

An Opportunity

The Chinese word "crisis" is composed of two characters meaning "danger" and "opportunity." This definition of crisis seems eminently fitting since it suggests a possible turning point for better or worse; it implies that we have the opportunity to correct unhealthy lifestyles and protect our future well-being and that of our children.

Dr. Jeffrey Koplan, former Director of the Centers for Disease Control and Prevention, began a lecture on bioterrorism with the statement that the major threats to our nation are obesity and sedentary lifestyle. What a powerful and thought-provoking statement!

As Dr. Stephen Bloom, of the Imperial College Faculty of Medicine, in London, says, "We've got a major epidemic sweeping the world, causing a massive increase in death." Dr. George Yancopoulos, Chief Scientific Officer and President of Regeneron Laboratories (Tarrytown, New York), further states that "obesity is the most dangerous epidemic facing mankind, and we are relatively unprepared for it." Drs. Jack and Susan Yanovski, of the National Institutes of Health, point out that "one of the most compelling challenges of the twenty-first century is to develop effective strategies to prevent and treat pediatric obesity."

Dr. Jeffrey Friedman, a leading obesity researcher at Rockefeller University and discoverer of leptin (a weight-regulating hormone), states, "Food consumes our interest. To the hungry, it is the focal point of every thought and action. To the hundreds of millions of obese and overweight individuals, it is the siren's song, a constant temptation that must be avoided lest one suffer health consequences and stigmatization. To the nonobese, it is a source of sustenance and often pleasure. To the food and diet industries, it is big business. And to those interested in public health, it is at the root of one of the most pressing public health problems in the developed and developing world."[4]

Hormonal changes may occur with loss of excessive weight; for example, ghrelin (called the "hunger hormone") may become elevated and increase appetite, whereas leptin, which ordinarily suppresses hunger, may decrease and thereby increase appetite. Unfortunately, these changes oppose efforts to lose weight. Whether leptin replacement has any role in combating obesity remains to be seen.

Evidence shows that a weight-reduced human body behaves metabolically and hormonally differently from a similar-sized body of a person who has not lost weight. After a person loses significant excess weight, muscles burn 20 to 25 percent fewer calories during ordinary activity or moderate aerobic exercise than muscles of persons at the same weight. How long these metabolic and hormonal changes remain after weight loss is not known, but they may persist for years. These findings provide a strong argument for preventing overweight and obesity and underscore the importance of teaching young children to eat healthy food and to exercise appropriately.

There is evidence that genetic factors program some individuals to consume more calories than others. For example, in an environment of food abundance, some gain weight while others do not. It is noteworthy that identical twins, even when separated and living in different households, maintain similar weights, while nonidentical twins usually have significantly different weights.

Genetic, hormonal, environmental, social, economic, and cultural factors are involved in the development of obesity; however, currently, to combat obesity by diet and exercise, we must depend on our behavior to control the amount of calories we consume and the amount of calories we burn up by physical activity.

How Much Should You Weigh?

Since 1960 the average weight of adult Americans has increased about 25 pounds, and the average dress size for women has increased from eight to fourteen. Unfortunately, the culture and environment in the United States encourage overeating and a sedentary lifestyle. In 1988 then Surgeon General C. Everett Koop correctly warned Americans that "one personal choice seems to influence long-term health more than any other: *what we eat.*"[5]

You can determine your approximate ideal weight from the table on the next page, the 1983 Metropolitan Life table showing desirable weight related to size of frame (body build), for ages twenty-five to fifty-nine, *in shoes with one inch heels and wearing five pounds of clothing for men, three pounds of clothing for women.* This table is helpful because it takes one's frame size into account. However, estimates of body weight for frame size and standard height-weight tables provide only a rough estimate of desirable weight, and they do not indicate whether a person is fat.

A more accurate way to learn whether your weight is excessive and might contribute to health problems is to determine your body mass index (BMI). BMI was developed as a tool to match body mass with risk for health problems; with most individuals it correlates with total body fat. However, it should be noted that an increased BMI does not always indicate increased body fat, since a muscular body may also increase BMI.

You can determine your BMI by dividing your weight in kilograms by the square of your height in meters (kg/m^2). If you prefer

Table 1. Height and Weight in Pounds Related to Body Size

MEN				WOMEN			
Height	Small	Medium	Large	Height	Small	Medium	Large
5′2″	128–134	131–141	138–150	4′10″	102–111	109–121	118–131
5′3″	130–136	133–143	140–153	4′11″	103–113	111–123	120–134
5′4″	132–138	135–145	142–156	5′0″	104–115	113–126	122–137
5′5″	134–140	137–148	144–160	5′1″	106–118	115–129	125–140
5′6″	136–142	139–151	146–164	5′2″	108–121	118–132	128–143
5′7″	138–145	142–154	149–168	5′3″	111–124	121–135	131–147
5′8″	140–148	145–157	152–172	5′4″	114–127	124–138	134–151
5′9″	142–151	148–160	155–176	5′5″	117–130	127–141	137–155
5′10″	144–154	151–163	158–180	5′6″	120–133	130–144	140–159
5′11″	146–157	154–166	161–184	5′7″	123–136	133–147	143–163
6′0″	149–160	157–170	164–188	5′8″	126–139	136–150	146–167
6′1″	152–164	160–174	168–192	5′9″	129–142	139–153	149–170
6′2″	155–168	164–178	172–197	5′10″	132–145	142–156	152–173
6′3″	158–172	167–182	176–202	5′11″	135–148	145–159	155–176
6′4″	162–176	171–187	181–207	6′0″	138–151	148–162	158–179

to use pounds and inches, divide weight in pounds by the square of your height in inches and then multiply by 703: [weight in pounds / (height in inches)^2] × 703 = BMI. For example, if you weigh 160 pounds and are 70 inches tall, then

$$\left(\frac{160}{70 \times 70}\right) \times 703 = \text{a BMI of about } 22.9.$$

You can also use the BMI calculator at www.nhlbisupport.com /bmi.

A BMI of 18.5 or less is considered underweight, 19 to 24.9 is judged healthy and desirable, 25 to 29.9 indicates overweight, 30 or over indicates obesity, and 40 or over is termed "morbid obesity,"

Table 2. Body Mass Index (BMI)

	Healthy		Overweight					Obese				
BMI	19	24	25	26	27	28	29	30	35	40	45	50
Height						Weight in pounds						
4'10"	91	115	119	124	129	134	138	143	167	191	215	239
4'11"	94	119	124	128	133	138	143	148	173	198	222	247
5'0"	97	123	128	133	138	143	148	153	179	204	230	255
5'1"	100	127	132	137	143	148	153	158	185	211	238	264
5'2"	104	131	136	142	147	153	158	164	191	218	246	273
5'3"	107	135	141	146	152	158	163	169	197	225	254	282
5'4"	110	140	145	151	157	163	169	174	204	232	262	291
5'5"	114	144	150	156	162	168	174	180	210	240	270	300
5'6"	118	148	155	161	167	173	179	186	216	247	278	309
5'7"	121	153	159	166	172	178	185	191	223	255	287	319
5'8"	125	158	164	171	177	184	190	197	230	262	295	328
5'9"	128	162	169	176	182	189	196	203	236	270	304	338
5'10"	132	167	174	181	188	195	202	209	243	278	313	348
5'11"	136	172	179	186	193	200	208	215	250	286	322	358
6'0"	140	177	184	191	199	206	213	221	258	294	331	368
6'1"	144	182	189	197	204	212	219	227	265	302	340	378
6'2"	148	186	194	202	210	218	225	233	272	311	350	389
6'3"	152	192	200	208	216	224	232	240	279	319	359	399
6'4"	156	197	205	213	221	230	238	246	287	328	369	410

Modified from National Institutes of Health Clinical Guidelines on the Identification, Evaluation and Treatment of Overweight and Obesity in Adults. 1998 *Mayo Clinic on High Blood Pressure*.

since it presents a serious health hazard. Table 2 will help you determine whether you are overweight or obese.

Determination of BMI in children requires the interpretation by a physician, since it depends not only on weight and height but also on gender and age. However, parents should become concerned if their child is significantly overweight and if the child develops abdominal obesity and requires oversized clothes compared to children of the same age.

The "Larding of America"

A few years ago we were the fattest nation in the world. Sixty-eight percent of adult Americans were overweight, and 34 percent were obese; 72.3 percent of men and 64.1 percent of women were overweight or obese. The incidence of obesity in the United Kingdom (22 percent), Germany (11.5 percent), France (9 percent), and Japan (3.2 percent) was significantly less. However, recently it was reported that in Finland, Germany, Greece, the Czech Republic, Slovakia, Mexico, Cyprus, and Malta, the proportion of overweight adults is greater than in the United States. The continuing bad news is that the percentage of obesity in Americans is still rising. In the United States 34 percent of women and 28 percent of men are obese; 6 percent of adult Americans are morbidly or super obese (one hundred pounds or more above ideal weight). In addition, obesity is more prevalent in Americans with low income. The increase in the incidence of obesity has been called the "larding of America." The number of obese adults has doubled in the past twenty years, and there is a pronounced weight gain with aging, as individuals become less active and have less muscle to burn up calories.

In addition, the number of overweight and obese children and adolescents in the United States has almost tripled since 1980. About seven years ago, more than 10 percent of children ages two through five, about 15 percent of children between six and eleven, and about 15 percent of teenagers were overweight, and almost 13 percent of children were obese. A more recent report reveals that in thirty states, 30 percent or more of children ages ten to seventeen were overweight or obese. Currently, it is estimated that about 32 percent of persons ages two to nineteen are overweight and 16 percent are obese.[6]

Furthermore, as mentioned in the last chapter, as early as three years old some obese children may have evidence of a type of inflammation linked to heart and blood vessel disease and hypertension in later life. To restate a point made in Chapter 1, intervention to prevent overweight and obesity in infancy and early childhood is essential. Excess maternal weight gain and smoking during pregnancy should be avoided, and an appropriate duration of breastfeeding is strongly recommended, since these steps may help prevent overweight and obesity in children and adults.

In the past decade type 2 diabetes has increased tenfold in children. It has been estimated that if obesity continues to escalate, of children born in 2000, 30 percent of Caucasians and 50 percent of African Americans and Hispanics will develop type 2 diabetes in their lifetime! Furthermore, elevated blood pressure may be 4.5 times more common in obese children than in those with normal weight, and sleep apnea occurs in one out of every ten obese children. If this increased trend toward obesity continues, life expectancy in this nation may indeed begin to decline in the near future by two to five years, and parents may live longer than their children. A recently introduced school program in Boston sends health report cards home to parents that detail information about student weight and physical fitness in an effort to get the attention of parents and enlist their help in combating childhood obesity.

It is particularly disturbing that some turnstiles at Disney World and some bus seats have been enlarged to accommodate obese individuals. Equally depressing is the marked increase in the demand for large coffins (forty-four inches across, compared with twenty-four inches for standard caskets), increased burial plot size (from three feet wide to four feet), and larger hearses. Most crematoria cannot accept bodies over five hundred pounds, and there is now a surcharge on embalming and transporting very obese individuals.

The main concern about overweight and obesity, of course, should be health and not appearance. At the same time, as mentioned, obesity can have a significant negative impact on the self-confidence and emotional health of children, adolescents, and adults. It can be a significant cause of peer rejection.

The Food Industry and Our Children

In her book *Food Politics,* Dr. Marion Nestle, professor and former Chair of the Department of Nutrition and Food Studies at New York University, depicts how the food and beverage industry has contributed to Americans' consumption of more calories. Much of the marketing has focused on foods high in fat and sugar and on soft drinks; the consumption of sodas has more than doubled in the past thirty years and is five times greater than it was fifty years ago. To promote greater sales and consumption, the food industry spends about thirty-three billion dollars yearly marketing its products, some of which is high in calories and low in nutrition ("junk food").

Sadly, success of this relentless food promotion correlates closely with increased obesity in the United States. Recently, food companies have targeted particularly vulnerable groups: children and members of minority groups. The result has been a progressive increase in caloric consumption and a steady fattening of America. Studies indicate that continually overeating appetizing junk food may trigger compulsive eating of calorie-rich food, similar to the addiction-like response in the brain caused by heroin. Most nutritional experts agree that "food preferences acquired in early childhood can endure throughout life, which could account for the ever-expanding American silhouette."[7]

Excessive weight and obesity, coupled with a sedentary lifestyle, are seriously impairing the health of our nation and, as mentioned above, are significantly adding to the skyrocketing cost of health care. Health care costs account for about 17 percent of the gross national product (GNP). The sensible dictum "Eat less and move more" has been relatively ineffective, and practiced only by a small percentage of the public. Research reports that children spend more time watching TV than engaging in other activities, and that they are exposed to twenty thousand commercials (about 150 to 200 hours) yearly. Unfortunately, most advertisements do not encourage eating healthy foods and rarely promote consumption of fruits and vegetables.

A sobering article recently reported that more than nine million young adults (27 percent of Americans ages seventeen to twenty-four) are too overweight to join the military.[8] Body weight is now the leading reason why recruits are rejected. Reversing this enormous health problem by every means possible is vital. Eliminating junk food, high-calorie beverages, and calorie-dense foods from school vending machines, and instilling a healthy lifestyle with healthy eating and appropriate physical activity are fundamental needs.

There is growing anger in some of the public who claim that certain fast-food restaurants are responsible for their obesity and the obesity of their children. However, this claim ignores the importance of parents' taking personal responsibility for their children's eating habits and with few exceptions has little merit. Increasingly, many fast-food businesses and restaurants are offering healthier foods and providing some guidance and information regarding calories, fat, and sugar content of their products.

Most public schools offer student lunches (paid for by the government) that contain reasonable nutrition. However, 20 percent of schools rely on money they receive from food and beverage companies to offset school budget cuts. In return, the schools permit sale of pizzas, burgers, and fries from some of the fast-food restaurants; many schools also have vending machines that dispense food, snacks, and soft drinks, often laden with fat and sugar. No school should have to depend on funds from restaurant chains that dictate the type of foods and drinks available to their "captive" students and staff. The unfortunate consequence is that most children and teenagers consume some foods and drinks high in calories that result in weight gain and obesity. Instead of sugary sodas, schools should make available bottled water, 100 percent fruit juice, and milk. As a nation, we literally are on a collision course to greater disease, disability, and death from lifestyle factors we can control. Fortunately, concern about marketing these foods and drinks to children has increased to the point that vending machines have been removed from the premises of many schools.

Persuading individuals to lose weight if they are not motivated to do so is very difficult, if not impossible. However, as touched on in Chapter 1, parental and teacher involvement may be especially helpful in encouraging some obese children and teenagers to eat healthful food and to exercise adequately. High-fat and high-sugar foods, cookies, candy, potato and corn chips, doughnuts, bakery products, crackers, sodas, and ice cream should not be readily available. Even low-fat foods usually contain a significant number of calories. A parent's example and efforts to help a child cope with any problem can sometimes be the key to success.

Food, or lack of food, releases hormones from the stomach, intestine, and fat cells that signal the brain and cause a person either to feel hungry and eat, or to feel full and stop eating. Although a genetic abnormality may account for some imbalance in these signals that could result in overeating, it appears that environmental and behavioral factors—especially excess consumption of solid fats (e.g., animal fats, butter, lard, hard cheeses) and products containing added sugars and refined grains, together with physical inactivity—play the major role in weight gain and obesity. Recent evidence links some genetic abnormalities with severe obesity in children. It has been said that "genes may load the gun, but environment pulls the trigger." Since we can't alter our genes, we must change our lifestyle to a program of healthy eating and physical activity. The duration and intensity of exercise have less of an effect on weight loss than the reduction of food and beverage calories.

However, adequate exercise maintains physical fitness and benefits cardiovascular function, which is more closely associated with longevity than body mass index (BMI) or waist circumference. It also increases muscle mass, which in turn helps to burn more calories. That the body needs less fuel with aging and that individuals usually become less active as they age partly explain an increase in body weight without any change in food or calorie consumption.

Finally, it is noteworthy that rapid weight gain and obesity are common side effects of antipsychotic and antidepressant medications used to treat young people and adults with mental disease.

Obesity's Link to Other Health Problems

If you are obese, your chance of developing hypertension may be eight times greater than that of normal-weight individuals. Obesity is the most important lifestyle factor causing or aggravating hypertension, which predisposes a person to, or aggravates, cardiovascular disease (hardening of the arteries, heart attack, heart failure, irregular heartbeat, stroke, and damage to vessels and retina of the eyes). Here are some statistics related to obesity and hypertension:

- Elevated blood pressure has been reported to be 3 to 4.5 times greater in obese than nonobese children and adolescents.[9]

- Hypertension occurs in approximately 50 percent of obese individuals.

- About 3 percent of children in the United States have hypertension, most of which is the result of obesity; another 10 percent are considered at risk for developing hypertension.

- About 30 percent of obese adolescents (eleven to nineteen years old) have hypertension.

Recent evidence indicates that obesity, even without hypertension, can strain the heart and cause it to enlarge and beat irregularly (atrial fibrillation). This may result in stroke, heart failure, and sometimes death. The occurrence of obesity in the very young may lead to the early development of heart and blood-vessel disease, such as hardening of the arteries (atherosclerosis) and other complications. Furthermore, recent evidence indicates that increased consumption of sugars used as sweeteners in processed foods can elevate harmful blood fats (LDL cholesterol and triglycerides) and lower the good HDL cholesterol; these changes can heighten the risk of stroke, heart disease, and hardening of the arteries.

Further consequences of obesity include impaired action of insulin and an increase in blood glucose levels, and an increase in harmful cholesterol and other unhealthy fats in the blood. These lead to the development of type 2 diabetes, heart disease, and hardening of the arteries. It is estimated that twenty-five million Americans have diabetes and almost sixty million have a tendency to develop diabetes. About 95 percent of people with type 2 diabetes are overweight or obese. Type 2 diabetes is uncommon in persons with a BMI below 22 (normal weight—see Table 2 on page 17), indicating that this type of diabetes may usually be prevented by maintaining a normal weight, even in individuals with a genetic predisposition to develop the disease. It is noteworthy that without adequate weight loss, type 2 diabetes usually becomes permanent after several years.

Overweight and obesity may also hasten the onset of type 1 diabetes, which occurs in children and young adults. Ninety percent of people with diabetes have type 2 diabetes, stemming from an inability of normal or even increased amounts of insulin to metabolize glucose normally. Type 1 diabetes results from an inadequate production of insulin by the pancreas. It is noteworthy that normally insulin is involved in carbohydrate, protein, and fat metabolism; however, in type 1 diabetes, the most important metabolic abnormality is insufficient insulin to maintain normal blood sugar concentrations.

One growing health concern is the development of nonalcoholic fatty liver disease, which affects up to 20 percent of American adults and has been linked to the occurrence of obesity. A small percentage of persons with this condition will develop liver inflammation with liver failure and cirrhosis or liver cancer. Other factors that may increase the risk of fatty liver disease are increased levels of harmful blood fats, the presence of type 2 diabetes, and consumption of some medications (e.g., steroids). Losing excess weight, adhering to a healthy diet, and increased physical activity can be beneficial.

Reduced lung capacity with impaired breathing, sleep apnea, gallstones, degenerative osteoarthritis (sometimes causing severe disability), varicose veins, blood clots, and hypertension in pregnancy are also not infrequent consequences of obesity. Recently, research has established that increased body weight is associated with higher death rates in men and women from cancers of the esophagus (swallowing tube), colon, rectum, liver, gallbladder, pancreas, kidney, and some malignancies involving the lymph tissue and bone marrow. Increased weight is also linked to higher death rates from stomach and prostate cancer in men, and from cancers of the endometrium (the lining of the uterus), cervix, ovary, and breast in women. Almost all common cancers are more frequent in the obese population and in persons with type 2 diabetes. It is estimated that overweight and obesity could account for 14 percent of all cancer deaths in men and 20 percent in women. Figure 1 on the following page demonstrates the percentage increase in the risks of various cancers as body mass index (a measure of body fat) increases.

Obesity makes surgery more difficult: Wounds do not heal as fast, and infections are more common. These medical problems can increase your doctor, medicine, and hospital bills. The considerably lower prevalence of obesity in the elderly is explained by the fact that most people who are significantly overweight die at a younger age than persons of normal weight.

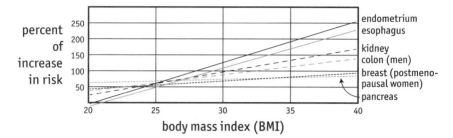

FIGURE 1. Increase in risk for certain cancers with higher body mass index (Source: Based on data from a 16 Feb. 2008 article in *Lancet*–Reprinted with permission from Mayo Foundation for Medical Education and Research. All rights reserved.)

Obesity is more strongly linked with chronic diseases than living in poverty, cigarette smoking, or alcohol consumption. Medical consequences and complications are burdensome for the obese population and increase the health-care costs for everyone else.

Metabolic Syndrome

Figure 2 shows the masterpiece Renaissance sculpture *David,* created by Michelangelo between 1501 and 1504. The seventeen-foot marble statue portrays the Biblical hero, probably immediately before his battle with Goliath. Figure 3 reveals what a modern American *David* might look like. This present-day David would be no match for Goliath.

Figures 4 through 6 on page 28 indicate the consequences of some of these complications. The combination of abdominal obesity, high blood pressure (greater than 130/85), type 2 diabetes or elevated blood sugar, elevated triglycerides (harmful blood fats), and decreased protective HDL cholesterol is known as metabolic syndrome. Metabolic syndrome exists if an individual has any three to five of these risk factors. (Originally this cluster of risk factors was given the title "deadly quartet." Sometimes, high triglycerides and low HDL are lumped together under the term "dyslipidemia," adding up to four factors rather than five.) In addition, individuals

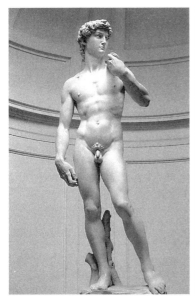

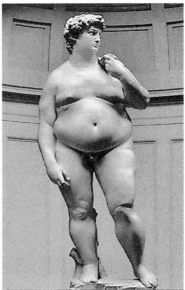

FIGURE 2. The ancient David

FIGURE 3. A modern American David

Some health conditions that may develop as a result of "American David's" obesity

Common Complications	Possible Complications
high blood pressure	Alzheimer's disease
stroke	impaired breathing and asthma
diabetes	cysts of the ovaries
many types of cancer	inflammation of the pancreas
osteoarthritis (knee and low-back pain)	varicose veins and blood clots
heart disease	altered hormone production
high bad cholesterol, low good cholesterol, high triglycerides	bone damage to legs
	infertility
hardening of arteries	difficult surgery
sleep apnea	pressure on the brain
acid reflux	fatty liver (sometimes hepatitis and cirrhosis)
	involuntary loss of urine
	hypertension in pregnancy
	gallstones
	gout
	low self-esteem and depression

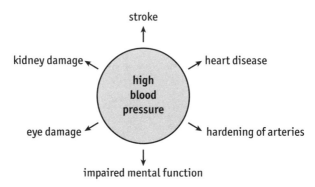

FIGURE 4. Conditions that may occur with high blood pressure

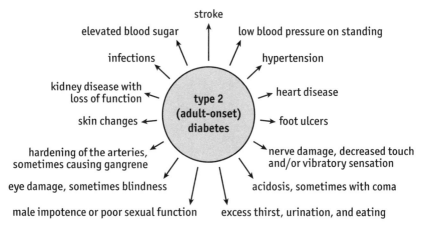

FIGURE 5. Conditions that may occur with type 2 diabetes

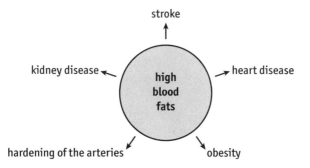

FIGURE 6. Conditions that may occur with high blood fats

with this syndrome tend to have high levels of C-reactive protein (CRP) in their blood, an indication of inflammation that may cause heart disease.

The metabolic syndrome is a major contributor to heart disease, stroke, hardening of the arteries, and kidney damage, even though individuals with this condition may not have a high level of harmful LDL cholesterol in their blood. Obese persons, especially Hispanics and African Americans, are particularly prone to developing metabolic syndrome. The good news is that losing as little as 10 percent excess weight may significantly reduce some or all of the abnormalities occurring in the metabolic syndrome.

We mentioned abdominal obesity as one of the conditions that make up metabolic syndrome. Why *abdominal* obesity? It turns out that the body shape of obese persons can be a predictor of health risk. Extra weight confined mainly to the waist, likened to an "apple-shaped" body, is associated with a higher risk for all the health problems caused by obesity. Researchers at Columbia Medical Center recently found that abdominal obesity was a greater risk factor for stroke in men and women younger than sixty-five than other risk factors (i.e., high blood pressure, diabetes, high harmful blood cholesterol, smoking, heart disease, alcohol consumption, and lack of exercise).

Why is this? Fat in the abdomen is metabolically very active, is released into the circulation, and can cause inflammation and arterial damage. A waist circumference (measured from the top of the pelvic bones around the waist) of more than forty inches in men, or thirty-five inches in women who are Caucasian, African American, or Native American is considered a health risk. For Asians, a waist circumference of more than thirty-six inches for men or thirty-two inches for women is a health risk. A simple rule to recall is that your waist circumference should measure no more than half the inches of your height. When weight is confined to hips and thighs, resulting in a "pear-shaped" body, a profile more commonly seen in women, there appears to be no greater health risk than in persons of normal weight. Fat in this area is thought to be metabolically inactive, is not released into the circulation, and does not cause arterial damage.

Recent statistics indicate that about 25 percent of adult Americans have metabolic syndrome, and roughly 50 percent over age fifty have it. Evidence suggests that obesity, particularly when associated with the metabolic syndrome, can impair intellectual function, memory, and learning ability of adolescents and adults. But even without metabolic syndrome conditions, obesity alone may cause heart failure.

The fact that obesity can lead to serious disease, disability, or death should convince the overweight or obese to start a program at once to lose excess weight. But despite a desire to lose weight, very few succeed unless firmly committed to do so.

Roger is an African American who recalls being obese when he was only twelve years old. At that time he was about five feet tall and weighed 195 pounds. A physical education program was not required in his school, and he rarely exercised; sports were not enjoyable because his weight markedly limited his ability to run and participate effectively as a team player. As a result, he usually spent six to seven hours daily watching TV from a couch, while constantly eating high-calorie snacks and drinking large amounts of sugar-laden sodas. Most of his meals consisted of fast foods with a high concentration of fat, few fruits and vegetables, and lots of sodas and ice cream. He always liked to add salt to his food.

Roger did not finish high school and continued to overeat and avoid any exercise except walking when necessary. By the time he was thirty, at five feet six inches tall he weighed 285 pounds. His blood pressure was very high (210/120), and it was discovered that he had type 2 diabetes and a very high level of harmful fats in his blood. This combination (abdominal obesity, diabetes, elevated blood fats, and hypertension)—indicating metabolic syndrome or the "deadly quartet"—is associated with a very high risk for cardiovascular disease. It was particularly important that he start medical treatment promptly and change to a healthier lifestyle.

Unfortunately, he delayed treatment until his eyesight became impaired as a result of hemorrhages and damage to the blood vessels and retina in the back of his eyes—the consequence of his hypertension and diabetes. He also experienced shortness of breath with even mild exertion, which resulted from enlargement of his heart and heart failure. By the time he finally began medical treatment his blood pressure and diabetes remained poorly controlled. At age thirty-five he suffered a massive stroke, which resulted in severe weakness of his right arm and leg, accompanied by impairment of his ability to talk distinctly.

Sadly, his physical limitations now prevent his working and supporting his wife and two young children. Had Roger maintained a normal weight, he probably would have avoided developing diabetes and the elevation of fats in his blood. He also may have avoided developing severe hypertension (although excess use of salt may increase blood pressure over time, particularly in salt-sensitive people). Today, with close medical management, his diabetes, blood pressure, and blood fats are under control, but the damage has been done.

· · · · · · · · ·

The combination of decreased calorie intake with increased calorie expenditure through greater levels of physical activity or aerobic exercise is essential for successful weight reduction. However, as we want to emphasize, the key ingredients for losing weight and maintaining weight loss are motivation and a commitment to a healthy lifestyle. For medical reasons, some individuals may be unable to increase their physical activity. But everyone has the ability to curtail overeating and combat this "hand-to-mouth" disease. Orson Welles, the late movie star and film director, confessed, "My doctor told me to stop having intimate dinners for four unless there are three other people." Unfortunately he did not follow his doctor's advice.

Changing from an unhealthy to a healthy lifestyle may do more than save your life. It may also have an enormous beneficial impact on your family—particularly your children. What could be more important than the health of your children? As mentioned in the Acknowledgments, the great humanitarian Albert Schweitzer said that "example is not the main thing in influencing others, it is the *only* thing." Parents should be good role models by choosing, preparing, and eating healthy foods and engaging in regular physical activity—and by doing so with their children whenever possible. Parental participation in helping their children discover a healthy lifestyle is extremely valuable. Your actions and lifestyle strongly influence those around you—especially young children. A noteworthy medical report in the *Archives of Family Medicine* revealed that children who dined with their family, if their family ate a healthful dinner, were more likely to eat nutritious food than if they were on their own.[10] Good parental example influences children to eat more vegetables and fruits, to drink more milk and fewer sodas, and to eat fewer fried, high-fat, and sugary foods. Improving your own health should be a basic desire. Benefiting the health of your children is an *obligation!*

3 ▶ **What** Are Americans Doing Wrong? (Or, Why Are We Fat and Getting Fatter?)

▶ Americans spend thirty billion dollars yearly trying to become and remain slim through various diets and exercise programs. Unfortunately, of those who lose weight, most regain the pounds they lost. This does not mean that one should not attempt to lose weight. Fortunately, modest weight loss of even ten pounds or 10 percent of body weight may lower blood pressure, blood sugar, and harmful (LDL) cholesterol.

The problem with most diet books is that they oversimplify a complex subject. In real life, there are thousands of food items to choose from, portion sizes are not standardized, and calories aren't the entire story—you also must contend with sugar, salt, and saturated fat. In addition, you need to know about the healthy components of a diet: vitamins, minerals, and antioxidants, to name just a few. Plus, what is thought to be important and healthy today might be proven to be less important and possibly not very healthy tomorrow. Consequently, many readers become confused and disinclined to spend the effort and time to prepare a diet schedule that will reduce their weight, lessen their hypertension, correct abnormal blood fats, and improve their diabetes. Some may lose interest and make no attempt to better their lifestyle unless the diet is easy to prepare and follow.

So, What Does Work?

It is most desirable to select a healthy eating plan that has been approved by the medical profession. The plan should be helpful in maintaining a healthy weight, and in controlling blood pressure, blood cholesterol, and type 2 diabetes. It should not require any special understanding of nutrition. The foods should be simple to prepare and delicious. (This list describes the DASH diet, which is explained in detail in the next chapter.)

Moderation in everything we do is central to our well-being and health. Overindulgence in high-calorie foods can be just as dangerous to your health as drinking excess alcohol or smoking. Overeating in general, but especially of high-calorie, high-fat foods and drinks—in combination with a sedentary lifestyle—will result in accumulation of excess body fat and weight gain. Genetic abnormalities may drive some to eat more without experiencing the normal sensation of being full after a meal. However, this should not interfere with your ability to lose weight if you are willing and committed to reduce your consumption of calories and if you increase the calories you burn with daily physical activity.

Our Fast-Food Habit

Many Americans are hooked on food prepared by the $129 billion fast-food industry, which continues to expand throughout the nation—just like Americans' waistlines, not coincidentally. It is estimated that more than half the money spent on fast food comes from drive-through business. That's why so many fast-food restaurants are adding drive-through facilities and are constantly seeking ways to deliver food more quickly. Many people, unwilling to be inconvenienced or to expend the energy to get out of their car, demand speedy service.

Often, restaurant meals contain more fat, cholesterol, and salt than home-cooked meals and are lower in calcium, potassium, and fiber. Adult Americans do not require more than 2,000 to 2,800 calories per day, unless they are very active. Unfortunately, many meals served in restaurants contain 1,500 to 2,000 calories *in a single meal*. Even some dinner plates have increased in size from 10½ inches to 12½ inches or larger.

Of great concern is the trend to offer larger servings of food and sodas ("super-sized" portions) at many fast-food restaurants. For example, in the mid 1950s, the combination of a hamburger, cola, and fries amounted to about 590 calories; today, a quarter-pound cheeseburger, super-sized fries, and super-sized cola are equivalent to 1,550 calories. A double hamburger with cheese, super-sized fries, and super-sized cola adds up to 2,050 calories—about as many calories as the average adult should consume in one day! The enormous growth since 1955 of serving sizes of three popular products is graphically illustrated in Figure 7.

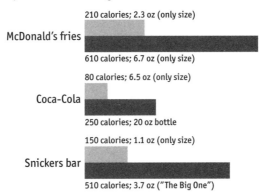

FIGURE 7. Monster portions: A graph showing how much serving sizes (by calories) of three well-known products have increased from 1955 to 2001. For children ages 7 to 10, nutritionists recommend a daily diet of 1,600 to 2,400 calories. (Source: Center for Science in the Public Interest)

A graphic illustration of how much sugar (about 7 teaspoons or 39 grams of carbohydrate) is contained in the standard 12-ounce can of Coca-Cola (Classic) is depicted in Figure 8 on the next page. It is estimated that the ordinary American diet may contain about 35 teaspoons of added sugar per day!

About 20 percent of calories consumed by Americans come from beverages. Very few adults and practically no children realize how much sugar is contained in even small-size sodas (see Figure 8 for a graphic reminder). Because soft drinks have very little nutritional value, they have been called "liquid candy." Sodas and sugar-sweetened beverages are reported to be "the single largest source of calories in the American diet"; 7.1 percent of the calories consumed in the United States are in the form of sugar-laden drinks.[1] It's an even greater proportion for young people: Sugared beverages now account for 10 to 15 percent of calories consumed by children and adolescents each day. Eating salty foods and snacks increases the desire to drink sodas, which further increases caloric consumption and weight gain. For each extra can or jumbo-sized serving of sugared beverage consumed daily, the likelihood of a child becoming obese increases by 60 percent!

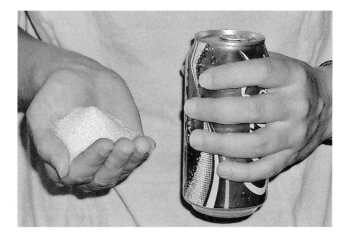

FIGURE 8. The amount of sugar in a 12 oz can of Coca-Cola (Source: dash forhealth.com)

An article in the *New York Post* compared the differences in food size and caloric content of three frequently eaten foods in the United States with those of the same foods in England and France (see Figure 9). The images dramatically illustrate the greater size and

caloric content of these popular foods when consumed "American style." (Of course, not everyone, even in the United States, regularly consumes a 20-ounce steak; the point of this illustration is to emphasize that in most other countries, such a large portion size wouldn't even be available.)

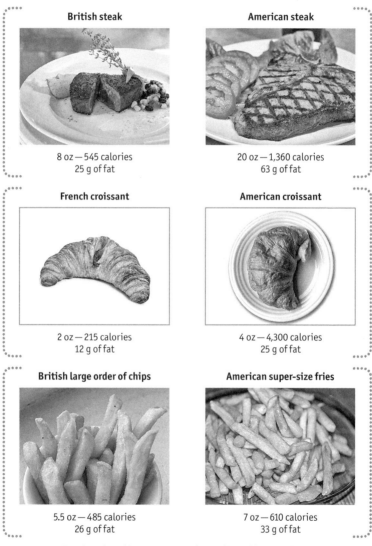

FIGURE 9. Portion sizes (Source: *New York Post/Page Six Magazine*, January 4, 2009; Courtesy of *The 9-Inch Diet* by Alex Bogusky, with modification)

The fast-food industry continues to offer super-sized portions. Furthermore, fast foods are becoming more available in schools in the United States; about 50 percent of school districts have contracts in place with soft-drink makers. Efforts are being made by some of the fast-food chains (e.g., McDonald's, Burger King, Subway, Pizza Hut, Taco Bell, Hardees, Kentucky Fried Chicken) to provide healthier food options and smaller portions with fewer calories. However, most of the public seem averse to changing their dietary habits significantly. Indeed, much more must be done to educate the public, particularly young children, to make the proper choices and follow a healthier eating plan. For example, most parents are unaware that chicken nuggets sold by fast-food chains contain about 57 percent of their calories from fat—almost twice the amount in an ordinary hamburger. Many young children regularly eat chicken nuggets, and this may result in a preference for fatty foods as they grow older. Chicken nuggets, currently very popular with both children and adults, can and should be prepared so that they contain mainly chicken and some carbohydrate but very little fat.

The downturn in the U.S. economy has increased the number and frequency of people eating the calorie-dense foods offered by the fast-food industry. Unfortunately, this further escalates the obesity crisis.

Liquid Calories

Figure 10 illustrates the rapid increase in the average daily calorie consumption in sodas from 1977 to 2001 in the U.S. In 1977 the amount of calories consumed daily from sodas was only 50, whereas between 1999 and 2001 the quantity increased to 150 calories. A recent publication from the Mayo Clinic indicated that the average American man, woman, and child each consumed more than fifty-two gallons of soda per year![2] The increase in calories from sodas has contributed to obesity and type 2 diabetes. Many states have banned or limited the sale of soft drinks in public schools, and some states are considering a tax on sugar-sweetened beverages to discourage consumption of these calorie-dense drinks.

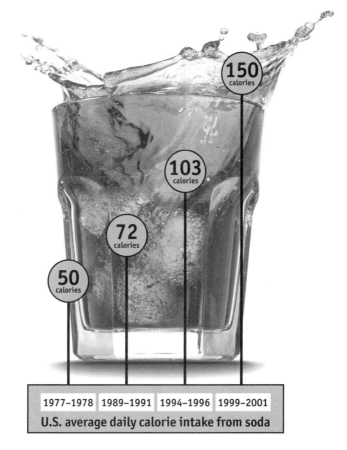

FIGURE 10. Average daily calorie intake from soda in the United States (Source: Courtesy of Mayo Clinic and Thinkstock)

Only "diet" sodas have no sugar added; instead, they usually contain aspartame, a harmless noncaloric sweetener. Other calorie-free sweeteners include Necta Sweet (saccharin), Sweet'N Low (dextrose, saccharin), Splenda (dextrose, maltodextrin, sucralose), and Equal (dextrose, maltodextrin, aspartame). All of these sweeteners appear to be harmless and are frequently added to tea and coffee. Most commercial brands of sweetened iced tea, lemonade, and fruit drinks similarly have a very high sugar content, and their use should be limited; instead, drink water or low-calorie ("diet") drinks more frequently. Of additional interest is a recent study that revealed that women who drank one or more sugar-laden sodas per day had an increase in the occurrence of gout, ordinarily quite rare in women; consumption of diet sodas, however, did not increase the occurrence of gout. A similar study in men revealed that consumption of five to six sugar-sweetened soft drinks per week increased the occurrence of gout compared to those who drank less than one soda per month.[3]

It is recommended that diet colas be decaffeinated, since excess consumption of caffeine can cause insomnia, nervousness, irritability, difficulty relaxing, anxiety, shakiness, and panic attacks. Caffeine can also temporarily increase the heart rate and cause heart irregularities. Black tea and green tea contain only one-quarter to one-half the amount of caffeine present in an eight-ounce cup of coffee. Tea is an excellent source of antioxidants, which are protective against a number of diseases. Furthermore, regular consumption of tea may be associated with higher bone density. (Herbal teas are not really teas but rather a combination of herbs, fruits, and spices.)

It is particularly worth mentioning that adding even light cream to one's coffee, over time, can add a very significant amount of calories. Figure 11 graphically illustrates this point; adding 4 ounces (½ cup) of light cream to coffee each day for just one month is equivalent to consuming about 7.6 sticks of butterfat, i.e., 7,100 calories per month! Most people don't add ½ cup of cream to their coffee all at once, but if you add 2 tablespoons per cup of coffee, and you drink four cups throughout the day, then you've consumed ½ cup of cream.

Dr. Thomas Moore, a major developer of the DASH eating plan, points out that using 4 ounces of half-and-half in your coffee

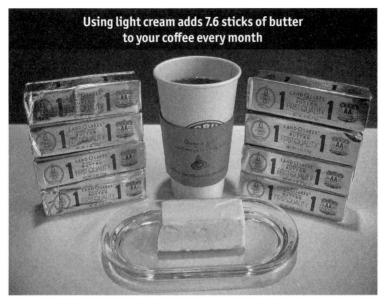

Using light cream adds 7.6 sticks of butter to your coffee every month

FIGURE 11. Adding 4 ounces of light cream to coffee every day for a month is equivalent to consuming about 7.6 sticks of butter, i.e., 7,100 calories per month. (Source: dashforhealth.com)

for one month is equivalent to 4.6 sticks of butterfat (4,700 calories), whereas using the same amount of whole milk is equivalent to 1.3 sticks of butterfat (2,400 calories). Switching from cream to whole milk in your daily coffee can save 4,700 calories in a month, which would add up to a weight loss of 1.3 pounds per month. As Dr. Moore points out, "Making small changes in one's diet can add up to big changes over time."

Be aware that many commercial iced coffee drinks contain coconut, chocolate, whipped cream, brownie pieces, and mocha syrup— and therefore, of course, a heavy load of calories.

Consumption of alcohol also adds extra calories with no nutritional value. There is evidence that a moderate intake of alcohol may be beneficial to some adults, especially those with coronary heart disease or type 2 diabetes. Moderation is defined as up to two drinks per day for men and up to one drink per day for women and for men age sixty-five or older. However, the data do not support recommending alcohol to persons who do not currently drink. A "drink" equals 12 fluid ounces of beer, or 5 ounces of wine, or 1½ ounces of hard liquor. Note that a cocktail may have added calories and other substances from the mixers; for example, tonic water contains high-fructose corn syrup and sodium.

Is there any wonder that weight gain seems inevitable, since so many Americans consume so many more calories than they should? It also is unfortunate that, as children, many of us were told to eat every bit of food on our plates. Many adults probably are conditioned to feel that eating everything on their plates is almost a duty. However, some restaurants permit ordering just half a portion of a food item. Ordering smaller portions or sharing full portions with a spouse or friend will save money and benefit your health by helping you to avoid excess calories. We should "eat to live—not live to eat"!

The Role of Dietary Fat

Many Americans eat far too much fat, often up to 40 percent of the calories in their diet. The dietary guidelines from the U.S. government recommend that adults get 20 to 35 percent of their calories from fat, with 10 percent from saturated fat and the rest from mono- and polyunsaturated fats. Fat comes mainly from meats and dairy products but can also be found in high quantities in some baked goods, salad dressings, chips, fries, and candy bars. Some very healthy fats are present in olive, canola, sunflower, and safflower oils, fish oils, avocados, and nuts. However, there is some evidence that when these "healthy" oils are used to fry foods, a toxic compound is produced that may be harmful to your health. Sources of unhealthy fats include animal fats, dairy products, nondairy creamers, shortening, some margarines, palm oil, and coconut oil.

Why does fat in the diet present a special problem? Every gram of fat has 9 calories, whereas every gram of carbohydrate or protein contains only 4 calories. Therefore, the same amount of fat supplies more than twice as many calories as carbohydrate or protein, and therefore, of course, is more fattening. A gram of alcohol affords 7 calories but no nutritional value. (See Chapter 4 for more about "good" dietary fats versus "bad" ones.)

In countries where individuals have traditionally eaten more fruits, vegetables, chicken, and fish—for example, in Greece, Italy, France, Spain, some Caribbean Islands, and many parts of South America and Asia—obesity was relatively rare in the past but is increasing. Some of the world's oldest people live in Greece and Japan. However, overweight has recently increased significantly in Greece, and longevity in Greece may decrease with complications of weight gain and obesity.

The Benefits of Calorie Restriction

When limited amounts of food are given to rats or mice in laboratory experiments, they live about 40 percent longer than when they are allowed to eat unlimited quantities of food. Lab monkeys also live longer—and healthier—when the amount of food they usually eat is reduced. Long-term studies have been conducted on rhesus macaque monkeys by lead researcher Richard Weindruch, associate scientist Ricki Colman, and others at the Wisconsin National Primate Research Center, at the University of Wisconsin, in Madison. They revealed that a nutritious but reduced-calorie diet (50 percent fewer calories) resulted in a lower weight and delayed the onset of age-related disorders such as cancer, type 2 diabetes, cardiovascular (heart and blood vessel) disease, and brain atrophy (decrease in brain tissue).

Monkeys on the lower-calorie diet also had a significantly longer life span than monkeys on the unrestricted diet. Over the course of the twenty-year study only 50 percent of the animals on the unrestricted diet survived, whereas 80 percent of animals on the restricted diet survived. A dramatic difference in the appearance of the monkeys on restricted and unrestricted diets is illustrated in Figures 12 and 13. These are particularly interesting results since this animal more closely resembles humans than other animals.

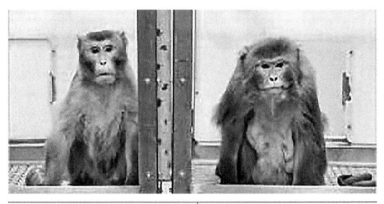

FIGURE 12. Canto, age 25, a monkey on a calorie-restricted diet of 445 calories per day (includes an apple each day).	**FIGURE 13.** Owen, age 26, a monkey on a normal diet of 885 calories per day (includes an apple each day).
Although a senior citizen—the average rhesus monkey lifespan in captivity is 27—**Canto**, above, is aging fairly well. Outwardly, he has a nice coat, elastic skin, a smooth gait, upright posture, and an energetic demeanor. His blood work shows he is as healthy as he looks.	He gets more food, but **Owen**, above, isn't aging as well. His posture has been affected by arthritis. His skin is wrinkled and his hair is falling out. Owen is frail and moves slowly. His blood work shows unhealthy levels of glucose and triglycerides.

(Credit: Courtesy Jeff Miller/University of Wisconsin–Madison)

Also noteworthy, in a separate experiment, is the finding of Dr. Sterling Johnson, a neuroscientist at the University of Wisconsin, that with aging an unrestricted diet was accompanied by loss of certain brain tissue (Figure 14) that governs mental and physical function.

The brain scan on the left shows the brain of a rhesus macaque allowed free rein at the dinner table (control), while the image on the right shows the brain of a monkey that for two decades was on a reduced-calorie diet (30 percent fewer calories). The brain of the animal allowed to eat freely has less tissue volume and more fluid (bright areas) than the brain of the monkey on the low-cal diet. The

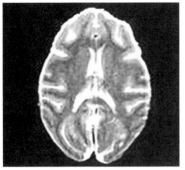 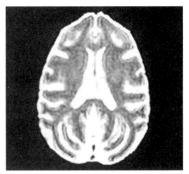

Brain scan of an animal on a
restricted-calorie diet

Brain scan of a control animal on an
unrestricted diet

FIGURE 14. Brain scans of monkeys (Credit: Courtesy Dr. Sterling C. Johnson)

images suggest less brain atrophy or cell loss with aging for animals that consume a diet with 30 percent fewer calories than if they were permitted to eat as much as they like. (Likewise, there is some evidence that aging in obese adult humans may be associated with decreased brain volume—atrophy—and a decline in brain function.) The studies on the rhesus monkeys are particularly noteworthy but require confirmation by others.

"Lean and less" is better for humans *and* animals. When food is restricted, body temperature and blood insulin levels are lowered, and the blood level of the steroid hormone cortisol remains steady—characteristics found in men who live the longest.

The China Study

Of particular interest is a book titled *The China Study* (2005), by world-renowned nutritionist T. Colin Campbell, PhD, and his son, T. M. Campbell, MD, in which they reported extensive studies of Chinese inhabitants living in rural communities. Body weights of the Chinese remained normal, and obesity did not occur. When compared with the usual American diet, it was found that 10 percent of protein consumed by the Chinese was obtained from animals, compared to 80 percent in the American diet. Furthermore,

Americans consumed more fat and cholesterol and less fiber than the Chinese. Although there has been some controversy surrounding the methodology of the authors' data gathering and statistical analysis, they make a strong argument that some cancers, type 2 diabetes, and hardening of the arteries are diseases of affluence, whereas diseases of poverty are more often linked to infections and parasitic diseases. They suggest that obesity is not significantly related to genetic abnormalities and that "we can control our obesity. It is right at the end of our fork." An equally amusing but sobering statement is the title of a book by former presidential candidate Mike Huckabee: *Stop Digging Your Grave with Your Knife and Fork.* Governor Huckabee was initially able to lose 110 pounds of excess weight with changes in his diet and exercise. Unfortunately, only a small percentage of persons who lose weight are able to maintain the weight loss, leading some to call the knife, fork, and spoon "weapons of mass destruction."

Recent surveys of adults in China reveal that heart disease there is skyrocketing; stroke remains about twice as common as heart attack. About 30 percent of the Chinese population have hypertension, 33 percent high cholesterol, 6 percent diabetes, and another 7 percent a tendency to develop diabetes. The cause of this increase in heart disease apparently is linked to the high prevalence of cigarette smoking, less exercise, and the increasing consumption of animal fats and fast foods, unavailable until recently. It was recently reported that Kentucky Fried Chicken now has over thirteen hundred restaurants in China. Trends in disease and unhealthy lifestyles are spreading to many developing countries.

Morbid Obesity and Weight-Loss Surgery

Compulsive eaters apparently derive gratification from eating excessively. Eating offers a comfort zone that relieves tension and anxiety. Many of these individuals may have emotional problems that are temporarily alleviated by overindulgence in food. In these persons the compulsive desire to eat may be viewed as somewhat similar to the cravings associated with alcoholism or smoking. For the compulsive eater, weight continues to increase, and some become morbidly obese, meaning that they weigh at least one hundred pounds above their ideal weight, occasionally as much as six times or more than normal healthy weight.

Obesity of this magnitude is a deadly condition that often results in the individual's being immobilized and bedridden because of the extreme effort and difficulty involved in walking or even changing positions. Very few hospitals have large enough wheelchairs, hospital beds, stretchers, operating tables, gowns, blood-pressure cuffs, weighing scales, or MRI and CAT machines to accommodate the markedly obese. Furthermore, excess fat frequently prevents images obtained by an MRI or CAT scan from being clear enough to see any injured areas or other abnormalities; excess breast fat also may interfere with accurate interpretation of mammograms. Even the average door width is often too narrow for the morbidly obese to pass through. These limitations—coupled with simple immobility— add further to the frustration, humiliation, depression, and misery of these individuals. Most people with morbid obesity develop hypertension, diabetes, and elevated harmful fats in their blood, and they die at a relatively young age from heart or kidney disease or stroke. Combating obesity in these individuals is extremely difficult. Special clinics exist to provide dietary treatment and emotional support to groups of these patients, which seem to be more effective than working with individual patients.

It has been found that weight-loss surgery, also known as bariatric surgery, works much better than medical treatment for mild type 2 diabetes in obese patients. Surgical procedures that bypass the stomach (gastric bypass surgery) decrease the amount of food absorbed. In addition, patients eat less food because they experience a rapid sense of fullness after eating even small meals. This potentially lifesaving surgery can cause marked weight loss that can be maintained. It is reported that blood sugar levels in about 80 percent of people with diabetes return to normal following bypass procedures. Diabetes may improve within days following gastric bypass, even before significant weight loss occurs, suggesting that changes in the intestine after bypass may improve diabetes, in addition to the eventual beneficial effect of weight loss. In addition to weight loss and improvements in diabetes, bariatric surgery usually markedly reduces excess fat in the liver and prevents liver inflammation and scarring.

Besides gastric bypass, a variety of bariatric surgical procedures are now available. Some reduce stomach size by wrapping an adjustable band around the upper part of the stomach, creating a small pouch above the band that makes patients eat less since they feel full after consuming a small meal. Following this type of stomach surgery, mild diabetes disappeared in 73 percent of patients, compared to only 17 percent of those treated medically.[4] Type 2 diabetes is a very serious health problem in the United States. Twenty-five million Americans have it, and almost sixty million are "prediabetic," that is, at risk for developing the disease. Because obesity is the major cause of type 2 diabetes, it is imperative to prevent or significantly reduce excess weight.

It is estimated that more than one hundred thousand morbidly obese Americans underwent bariatric surgery in 2004—about four times as many as in 1998—and enthusiasm for the procedure continues to grow. On the downside, bariatric surgery can be very difficult, especially when obesity is very marked, and it has been reported that one of every fifty patients dies from complications of the operation. Therefore, it is extremely important to have bariatric surgery performed at a medical center where surgeons have done a large number of the procedures and have developed special expertise. It is also critical that a medical team supervise the patient's progress after surgery in order to avoid the numerous complications that can occur. There is currently uncertainty about the long-term outcomes of bariatric surgery. Benefits appear independent of weight loss.

Obesity and Pregnancy

Of considerable concern is a recent report that today about half of the women of childbearing age are overweight or obese. Excess weight and obesity of expectant mothers may increase the risk of preeclampsia (high blood pressure in pregnancy), birth defects, fetal deaths, and preterm delivery. The need for Caesarean section rather than natural-birth delivery has progressively increased. Excess weight before pregnancy and excess weight gain during pregnancy also are associated with fatter babies, who often are destined to become fatter adults. The Institute of Medicine recommends that during pregnancy thin women can gain 28 to 40 pounds, normal-weight women 25 to 30 pounds, overweight women 15 to 25 pounds—and obese women no more than 11 to 20 pounds. Sadly, about 60 percent of pregnant women gain more than these recommended amounts.

Some physicians now recommend that very obese women undergo bariatric surgery before becoming pregnant to decrease the risks associated with childbearing. Bottom line: It is particularly important for women who may become pregnant or for those already pregnant to avoid excess weight. It is also recommended that women breastfeed their babies, since breastfed children may be at less risk for developing overweight or obesity than those who are bottle-fed.

The Dangers of Diet Pills

Drugs that reduce the desire to eat or that decrease the amount of fat absorbed from the intestine are not usually very helpful and may cause undesirable side effects. Such drugs should be used only under the direction of a physician, and only in conjunction with a healthy diet and regular exercise.

Dietary supplements and products containing ephedra (ma huang), ephedrine, or phenylpropanolamine for weight loss should never be taken. They can stimulate the nervous system, markedly elevate blood pressure and heart rate, and may occasionally cause heart attack, stroke, or death. Initially, the American Medical Association and the American Heart Association urged that all ephedra supplements be banned; its use was then banned by the National Football League, and its use by athletes in college competition and in the Olympics was prohibited. Unfortunately, professional baseball, basketball, and hockey teams did not make every effort to prevent the serious health consequences of this very dangerous drug. However, in December 2003 the Food and Drug Administration (FDA) announced that sale of supplements containing ephedra would become unlawful. Later, the ban on ephedra was lifted to permit low doses to be used. Despite these efforts, ephedra probably played a role in the 2003 death of twenty-three-year-old Baltimore Orioles pitcher Steve Bechler, who collapsed during a workout and died the next day. Over one hundred deaths have been reported in persons taking ephedra, and numerous episodes of brain damage (strokes), seizures, heat stroke, heart attack, and mental changes (psychosis) have been reported.

Other supplements are available that are supposed to increase metabolism and burn fat. An article in *The New York Times* on March 4, 2003, recounted the frightening experience of Jennifer Rosenthal, a twenty-eight-year-old California mother. She was not overweight but "just wanted to stay in shape."[5] A friend recommended that she take capsules containing usnic acid, which is supposed to increase metabolism and burn fat. Rosenthal started taking half the maximum dose of the capsules; about a month later, she was in a coma and on a respirator, and her skin turned a dusky yellow. Fortunately, a liver from a cadaver became available and was transplanted to replace her own severely damaged liver, which had shrunk to about one-third its normal size. Without this transplant she would have died in a few days. She is currently taking many medications, some of which are essential to prevent rejection of the transplanted liver. She will have to continue some medications and limit her activities for the rest of her life.

It is extremely important to be aware that some dietary supplements (products of herbs and plants) may be very harmful or fatal. Unfortunately, these substances are unregulated and are easily purchased in food stores and over the Internet. Many are obtained from foreign countries and may contain harmful ingredients. You should never use supplements if their safety and effectiveness are unknown, since they can be both dangerous to your health and ineffective for weight loss. Always ask a physician when considering the use of a supplement. It has been reported that about $24 billion was spent on dietary supplements in 2007, $1.7 billion of it for weight-loss pills. Furthermore, according to the Centers for Disease Control and Prevention, about 15 percent of Americans said they had used weight-loss supplements, and most had not reported doing so to their doctors.[6]

. . . .

Former U.S. Surgeon General David Satcher stated, "Being overweight or obese may soon cause as much preventable disease and death as tobacco." Dr. Mark Jacobsen of the American Academy of Pediatrics has suggested that the cost of obesity-related diseases may outstrip the health-care costs of cigarette smoking. American physicians, some obese themselves, are aware of the dangerous consequences of obesity, and they should strive to educate their patients about its seriousness. More attention should be paid to educating physicians, medical students, and other health-care providers regarding the importance of proper nutrition, exercise, and weight control for patients. Furthermore, the government and local communities can help raise the level of awareness of the health risks of obesity. Educating the public about the seriousness of obesity and related diseases that can be prevented, or at least controlled, is essential to saving many lives.

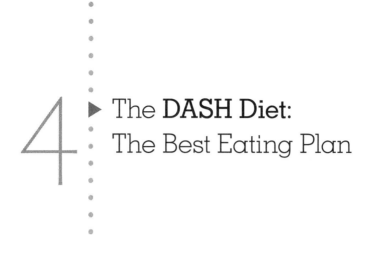

4

▶ The **DASH** Diet: The Best Eating Plan

▶ Fortunately, there is a dietary plan that has been physician-approved. It's called the DASH eating plan. "DASH" stands for Dietary Approaches to Stop Hypertension. As the name implies, it was originally developed to treat high blood pressure, but it has been recognized as a very beneficial eating plan overall—both for healthy people who want to maintain their well-being and for those who want to lose weight and/or improve their cardiovascular health.

Whenever you want to make a major life change, such as adopting healthier behaviors that will lead to weight loss, you need to educate yourself about both the *what* and the *how*. In the case of weight reduction, that means learning not only *what* to eat, but also *how* to incorporate the changes into your everyday life so they become lifelong habits. (Of course, there is a bit of overlap between the two topics.) This chapter focuses on the *what,* and the next chapter focuses on the *how*.

Characteristics of a Healthy Eating Plan

A healthy eating plan has several characteristics, outlined below. The DASH diet encompasses all of these features.

It will help you reduce your weight to an acceptable range and maintain it there (refer to BMI in Table 2 on page 17).

It includes foods (particularly lots of fruits and vegetables— fresh, frozen, canned, or dried) that are high in potassium (which tends to lower blood pressure and prevent strokes), other minerals, vitamins, antioxidants, and fiber.

It limits percentage of daily calories from dietary fat to 30 percent or less, and it especially decreases calories from saturated fat to 10 percent or less. It also limits dietary cholesterol. These changes will lower "bad" (LDL) cholesterol and triglycerides in the blood.

It includes low-fat or nonfat dairy foods, which are major sources of calcium and protein.

It limits daily consumption of meat and poultry (without the skin) to no more than two 3-ounce servings (6 ounces total). Eating a variety of fish, at least twice a week, as a major source of protein, is recommended. However, fish that may contain mercury (particularly fatty fish, e.g., swordfish, shark, king mackerel, tilefish, and albacore tuna) should be limited to no more than once weekly and avoided by pregnant women, women of childbearing age, and nursing mothers. Although shellfish, such as shrimp and lobster, have a moderate amount of cholesterol, they have very little fat and are low in calories. They may be eaten occasionally if not prepared or soaked with butter. Avoid fried fish and poultry, especially batter-dipped or breaded. Persons with a history of gout should avoid excess consumption of foods high in purine, e.g., mackerel, herring, sardines, roe (i.e., fish eggs), anchovies, scallops, mussels, organ meats, meat extracts, consommé, gravy, shellfish, and other purine-rich foods.

It limits sugar and "junk" foods (sodas, chips, candy bars, etc.), which are high in calories and low in nutritional value. Carbohydrates provide the major energy source for the body, and they consist of two types: starches and sugars. The body converts these to glucose, which provides energy. Glucose is especially important for brain function. Starches are abundant in breads, pastas, rice, potatoes, and vegetables, whereas sweet-tasting foods, with the exception of fruits in their natural form, usually contain added sugars—e.g., candy, cookies, ice cream, sodas, some fruit juices, and sweetened dairy products. There is considerable concern that high-fructose corn syrup, which sweetens many soft drinks and some foods, may have undesirable effects, such as increasing triglycerides and uric acid in the blood. Furthermore, fructose (the sugar found in honey and in fruit), which is metabolized in the liver, may cause a fatty liver and may impair the liver's function. It can also cause weight gain. Finally, an excessive intake of sugar and other refined carbohydrates can elevate levels of triglycerides in the blood.

It helps lower elevated blood pressure by limiting total salt intake to no more than 5.8 grams (about one teaspoon) daily (equivalent to 2,300 milligrams of sodium). For most Americans, limiting salt intake to 3.0–3.8 grams (equivalent to 1,200–1,500 milligrams of sodium) is even better, especially for African Americans and those with hypertension, diabetes, and/or impaired kidney function. The one teaspoon includes *both* salt in processed food *and* salt used in cooking and at the table. It is especially important to learn to read food labels and become aware of foods that have a high concentration of sodium, total fat, saturated fat, cholesterol, and added sugar so that you can limit them. (See Chapter 9, "The Salt Story.")

It limits alcohol consumption to no more than two drinks of wine, beer, or spirits per day for men and one drink per day for women.

It includes foods high in fiber, such as whole-grain cereals and breads, fruits, vegetables, and legumes (all types of beans, peas, and lentils). Surprisingly, coffee also contains fiber. There are two forms of fiber—soluble and insoluble. Soluble fiber dissolves in water; insoluble fiber, which does not dissolve, provides bulk to the stool and promotes regular bowel movements. Increasing fluid consumption can help prevent the constipation sometimes caused by adding fiber to the diet. Fiber is a complex carbohydrate and provides no calories, since it is not digested by the body. Soluble fiber can reduce bad (LDL) cholesterol and sugar in the blood, and it may decrease hunger and reduce weight; it appears to play a beneficial role in reducing the risk of heart disease, diabetes, and colon and breast cancer. It is recommended that adults eat about 25 to 30 grams of fiber daily. Children should aim for 5 grams plus their age in grams. Fruits and vegetables and their skins (if edible) are particularly abundant and healthy sources of fiber. If desirable, you can increase soluble fiber intake by taking a fiber supplement such as Metamucil.

It includes adequate dietary calcium (up to 1,500 milligrams daily for adults, depending on age and gender) and adequate vitamin D (usually about 400 IU daily). Vitamin D helps the body absorb calcium. Some vitamin D is produced in the skin by exposure to sunlight, but the elderly and those not exposed to sunlight may require in intake of up to 800 IU. A blood test can determine if you have adequate vitamin D in your body. Both calcium and vitamin D are important in preventing and treating osteoporosis. Some fruit juice, milk, and foods are fortified with calcium and vitamin D; however, supplemental calcium and vitamin D may be needed. Supplemental calcium and vitamin D should not be consumed by those who have had calcium stones in their urinary tract.

It includes adequate vitamins and minerals (in addition to the ones already mentioned in this section, i.e., potassium, calcium, vitamin D). Although the body cannot make vitamins (A, C, D, E, K, B_6, B_{12}, thiamin, riboflavin, niacin, folic acid, biotin, choline, and pantothenic acid) or minerals (sodium, potassium, calcium, magnesium, manganese, copper, iodine, fluoride, iron, phosphorus, chloride, chromium, selenium, molybdenum, and zinc), severe deficiencies of these substances are uncommon in the United States if people are in good health and are eating a balanced diet with a variety of nutritious foods. However, many adults, particularly the elderly, persons who are chronically ill, and those who do not eat a balanced diet, may have a mild deficiency of some vitamins, especially vitamins D and B_{12}. Individuals on "crash" or "fad" diets and strict vegetarians can develop vitamin and mineral deficiencies, which require adding appropriate amounts of the deficient vitamins and/or minerals to the diet. Crash diets should not be used to lose weight, since they can be hazardous to your health. (See Chapter 6 for a brief summary of some popular weight-loss diets.)

It is enjoyable and easy to follow. This will help people stick to it.

Vitamins and Minerals: A Few Recommendations

It is worth noting a few important guidelines about some specific vitamins and minerals. An estimated 40 percent of the U.S. population does not consume adequate folic acid (folate). Women of childbearing age should consume 400 micrograms of folic acid daily (which is contained in most multivitamin pills). Supplementing with folic acid can markedly decrease the risk of a certain type of nerve defect in babies. Folic acid may also be beneficial by reducing blood levels of a substance called homocysteine, high levels of which have been associated with hardening of the arteries. (Most recently it has been reported that reducing blood homocysteine does not reduce heart disease.)

Menstruating women should consume adequate dietary iron to avoid the possibility of iron-deficiency anemia. Pregnant women should follow the diet and take the dietary supplements prescribed by their health-care provider. (As an aside, it is noteworthy that breastfeeding appears to afford a protective effect against the development of obesity in a woman's offspring. Moreover, mothers who breastfeed may return to pre-pregnancy weight more quickly than those who bottle-feed their babies.)

Bottom line: For those who do not eat a balanced diet with a variety of foods, to avoid deficiencies, it seems reasonable to take a one-a-day vitamin/mineral supplement that provides 100 percent of the recommended daily values.

Megadoses of vitamins should be avoided or taken with caution and with a physician's advice, since some of them can cause serious side effects. There is no convincing evidence that large doses of vitamin C prevent infections, cancer, or any other disease. High doses of vitamin C may sometimes cause kidney stones. A high intake of vitamin A has been associated with an increased risk of hip fracture in postmenopausal women and with fetal abnormalities during early pregnancy. Very high doses of vitamin A and beta-carotene (which the body converts to vitamin A) may increase the occurrence of lung cancer (particularly in smokers and workers exposed to asbestos) and may also increase death from heart and blood vessel damage. Increased consumption of some minerals can also be dangerous; again, you should always consult a physician before taking megadoses of any nutrient.

Dietary Cholesterol and Dietary Fats

It is worth discussing dietary fats and cholesterol in some detail because they play such a large role in overall health and weight control. Elevated blood levels of "bad" (LDL) cholesterol and probably of triglycerides (fats) increase the risk of heart attack, stroke, and hardening of the arteries. All adults, even those with normal blood cholesterol and triglycerides, should have their blood work done about every five years to detect any abnormalities in what's called the lipid profile (measurement of these cholesterol and triglyceride levels). It is especially important to check a person's blood for abnormalities if any family member has elevated harmful cholesterol or triglycerides, or if there is a family history of heart attack or stroke at a young age. Children also should be tested for elevated cholesterol and triglycerides at age ten so that appropriate treatment may be implemented if indicated. In the presence of hypertension the risk of these complications is significantly greater, which makes it even more important to reduce the level of "bad" fats in the blood in addition to normalizing blood pressure.

Dietary choices and body weight can have a major effect on a person's blood lipid profile. The first thing is to be aware of foods that contain cholesterol and harmful fats, particularly saturated fats and trans fats (described below). Be aware that processed foods claiming to be "low fat" may still be high in calories and therefore undesirable for those trying to lose weight. The rest of this section takes a closer look at dietary cholesterol and dietary fats.

Dietary Cholesterol

Cholesterol is necessary to the body. Produced in the liver, it is involved in important functions such as the production of bile (a substance that helps to break down dietary fats) and maintaining the flexibility of cell walls. Besides being manufactured by the human body, cholesterol is found in foods of animal origin—meat, dairy products, and eggs. Foods high in cholesterol include:

- egg yolks
- shellfish
- meats (especially organ meats)
- dairy products, especially those made with whole milk (butter, ice cream, whipping cream, heavy cream, half and half, cheese, yogurt; low-fat and fat-free dairy products have less cholesterol)

Since your body already produces adequate cholesterol, you should limit its consumption. Cholesterol does not provide calories, but, as stated, increased amounts of "bad" cholesterol (LDL) can damage and clog the arteries. Eggs are a good source of digestible protein, yet they contain high amounts of cholesterol (about 210 milligrams per egg yolk). It now appears that eating six or fewer eggs per week may not be harmful and does not increase the risk of heart attack and stroke *in persons who are in good health*. However, in individuals with diabetes, increased blood cholesterol, and/or cardiovascular disease, excess consumption of egg yolks may elevate cholesterol levels and increase the risk of heart attack and stroke; such individuals should limit dietary cholesterol to less than 300 milligrams daily. It is noteworthy that the way individuals handle the cholesterol they consume may differ markedly. In some individuals much more dietary cholesterol is absorbed and may result in high levels of harmful LDL, whereas in others relatively small amounts of dietary cholesterol are absorbed with little formation of LDL cholesterol.

Saturated Fats

Saturated fats raise the bad cholesterol (LDL), increase the risk of heart attack and stroke, and contribute to insulin resistance. Saturated fats include:

- animal fats (contained in meat, poultry, fish), lard (pig fat), and full-fat dairy products (butter, cream, whole milk)
- milk chocolate and white chocolate, cocoa (cocoa powder is acceptable; in limited amounts, dark chocolate may be beneficial, since it has antioxidants and should not increase the risk of heart attack and stroke)
- coconut oil and palm oil (often used in baked goods)

Saturated fats, like all fats, are also high in calories and should be very limited or avoided when possible, especially in those who are overweight or obese and trying to lose weight.

Trans Fats (Trans Fatty Acids)

Trans fats, also known as hydrogenated vegetable oils, are partially saturated fats artificially prepared from unsaturated fats by adding hydrogen to vegetable oils to solidify the oil and increase its shelf life. Very few trans fats occur naturally. Trans fats are even more unhealthy and harmful than naturally occurring saturated fats, and they increase the risk of heart attack and stroke. They *increase* bad cholesterol (LDL) and triglycerides in the blood. They *decrease* good cholesterol (HDL) in the blood.

In the past, trans fats were often found in:

- some margarines
- shortening (fat)

These fats are used to make:

- French fries
- tortillas
- doughnuts
- multigrain cereal bars
- pie crusts
- fried chips
- pudding
- crackers
- cookies and bakery products
- nondairy creamer

Currently most of these foods are available in supermarkets and do not contain trans fats. Sometimes, however, a few of these food items still contain trans fats, so read your food labels carefully.

Under FDA rules, food labels must indicate the amount of trans fats contained in foods, unless the amount is very small. If the ingredient list of a food label contains hydrogenated fats, then a small amount of trans fats is present. Newer varieties of margarine contain no trans fats and are low in saturated fat. Several margarines (e.g., Smart Balance, Take Control, and Benecol) lower the LDL cholesterol. Olive oil is a healthful substitute for butter or margarine. It can lower LDL, but, like all fats and oils, it is higher in calories than proteins and carbohydrates.

Monounsaturated Fats

Whenever possible, replace trans fats with monounsaturated fats. They are found in:

- olive oil
- peanut oil
- canola oil
- avocados
- some nuts (e.g., almonds, cashews, hazelnuts, pecans, walnuts)

These healthy fats tend to lower LDL cholesterol and do not damage arteries. People in Spain, France, Italy, and Greece—who tend to consume fat in the form of olive oil, eat lots of vegetables, fruits, and whole grains, and eat smaller portions of meat and processed foods (known as the "Mediterranean diet")—have lower rates of heart disease. Adhering to the Mediterranean diet, which is very similar to the DASH diet, can reduce death from cardiovascular disease and the occurrence of and death from cancer. This diet may also reduce the incidence of Parkinson's and Alzheimer's disease and brain damage from small strokes. Furthermore, combining regular exercise with the Mediterranean diet can reduce the risk of developing Alzheimer's disease by 48 percent.

Polyunsaturated Fats

Saturated and trans fats can also be replaced with polyunsaturated fats, which include the following:

- corn oil
- sunflower oil
- safflower oil
- cottonseed oil
- soybean oils
- omega-3 fats (contained in fish, soy, and flax oil)

These are far healthier than saturated fats and may lower LDL cholesterol. Nevertheless, they can produce changes in the body that can damage arteries; also, excessive use of any oil can add significant calories and promote weight gain.

If weight loss (when indicated), exercise, and healthy nutrition do not sufficiently lower the LDL cholesterol and triglycerides, then medication may be necessary and should be prescribed by a physician.

Protein

Limiting the percentage of protein in your diet is not recommended for weight reduction. A healthy diet should contain 15 to 20 percent of calories from protein. The Atkins diet increases protein intake to 30 percent of calories to replace the marked reduction of carbohydrate; however, a diet high in protein is difficult for most persons to consume for a prolonged time and can be detrimental to persons with some kidney or liver diseases. (See Chapter 6 for more on the Atkins diet and other popular weight-loss programs.) Protein is an important source of energy and is essential to building muscles and organs in the body. It is plentiful in many foods, especially meats, poultry, fish, shellfish, nuts, dairy foods, eggs, and beans. However, it is best to eat less meat and to trim and remove as much fat as possible from beef, lamb, veal, venison, and pork; skin of poultry should be removed and not eaten because of its fat and cholesterol content.

Egg whites contain only protein (as do Egg Beaters) and are very nutritious. They don't contain any cholesterol, which is found only in the egg yolk. Another good source of protein is soy. Soy foods come in many forms and are a rich source of a form of protein that may lower LDL cholesterol.

The DASH Diet

The Dietary Approaches to Stop Hypertension (DASH) eating plan is outlined in Table 3 on the next page. The foods included in DASH can be easily prepared and are tasty and healthy. This eating plan has been recommended as an *extremely healthy eating plan for nearly all*

Americans by the American Heart Association, the United States Department of Agriculture, the National Cancer Institute and National Heart, Lung and Blood Institute of the National Institutes of Health, the National Hypertension Association, 2010 Dietary Guidelines for Americans, leading medical centers, and many registered dietitians. Most health and nutrition experts agree that the DASH eating plan is the healthiest ever recommended.

Table 3. The DASH Eating Plan (based on about 2,000 calories per day)

Food Group	Daily Servings	Serving Sizes	Examples	Significance to the DASH Diet
Grains and grain products	7–8	1 slice bread ½ C* dry cereal ½ C cooked rice, pasta, or cereal	Whole-wheat bread, ½ English muffin (small), pita bread, bagel, cereals, grits, oatmeal (Typical bagel = 4 servings of grains)	Major sources of energy and fiber
Vegetables	4–5	1 C raw leafy vegetable ½ C cooked vegetable 6 oz vegetable juice	Tomatoes, potatoes, carrots, peas, squash, broccoli, turnip greens, collards, kale, spinach, artichokes, beans, sweet potatoes	Rich sources of potassium, magnesium, and fiber
Fruits	4–5	6 oz fruit juice 1 medium fruit ¼ C dried fruit ½ C fresh, frozen, or canned fruit	Apricots, bananas, dates, oranges, grapefruit, mangoes, melons, peaches, pineapples, prunes, raisins, strawberries, tangerines	Important sources of potassium, magnesium, and fiber
Low-fat or nonfat dairy foods	2–3	8 oz milk 1 C yogurt 1½ oz cheese	Skim or 1 percent milk, skim or low-fat buttermilk, nonfat or low-fat yogurt, part-skim mozzarella cheese, nonfat cheese	Major sources of calcium and protein
Lean meat, poultry, fish Eggs**	2 or fewer 6 or fewer per week	3 oz cooked meat, poultry, or fish	Select only lean meat; trim away visible fats; broil, roast, or boil instead of frying; remove skin from poultry. (Can also be grilled.)	Rich sources of protein and magnesium

(cont'd.)

Table 3. The DASH Eating Plan (based on about 2,000 calories per day) (cont'd.)

Food Group	Daily Servings	Serving Sizes	Examples	Significance to the DASH Diet
Nuts, seeds, legumes	4–5 per week	1½ oz or ⅓ C nuts, ½ oz or 2 Tbsp seeds ½ C cooked legumes	(Unsalted) almonds, filberts, mixed nuts, peanuts, walnuts, sunflower seeds, lentils, kidney beans	Rich sources of energy, magnesium, potassium, protein, and fiber
Fats and oils	2–3	1 tsp soft margarine, vegetable oil, or butter, 1 Tbsp regular fat mayonnaise or salad dressing 2 Tbsp low-fat or nonfat salad dressing or mayonnaise	Soft margarine, low-fat mayonnaise, light salad dressing, vegetable oil (such as olive, corn, canola, or safflower)	Source of essential fatty acids, minor source of energy
Sweets	5 per week	1 Tbsp sugar 1 Tbsp jelly or jam ½ oz jelly beans 8 oz lemonade	Maple syrup, sugar, jelly, jam, fruit-flavored gelatin, jelly beans, hard candy, fruit punch, sorbet, ices	Sweets should be low in fat. Minor source of energy

(Source: "Dietary Approaches to Stop Hypertension" (DASH), the Sixth Report of the Joint National Committee, November 1997. [The DASH Diet–NIH publication 01-4082. Revised May 2001]. Slight modifications in parentheses for clarity.)
* C = cup
** Added eggs to DASH diet. Note: no more than six egg yolks per week; egg whites do not have to be limited. Persons with diabetes or high LDL cholesterol and/or cardiovascular disease should eat eggs only occasionally (three or fewer per week).

Here is a summary of the main features of the DASH eating plan:

- It is lower in fat (about 27 percent of calories) than the typical American diet, especially saturated fat.
- It is rich fruits and vegetables (four to five servings *of each* daily).
- It features low-fat or nonfat dairy products.
- It emphasizes whole grains over refined (white) ones.
- It is low in dietary cholesterol.

- It is high in fiber, potassium, calcium, and magnesium.
- It is moderately high in protein, focusing on nuts, seeds, and legumes (peas, beans, and lentils) to provide healthy protein, and allowing smaller but adequate amounts of meat, fish, and poultry.

Figure 15 displays a proposed pyramid for DASH foods. This pyramid differs from other well-known pyramids by emphasizing more servings of fruits and vegetables and less consumption of meat, poultry, and fish. However, the recently proposed Mayo Clinic Healthy Weight Pyramid is quite similar and permits consumption of unlimited amounts of healthful fruits and vegetables, since there is only a small amount of calories in large amounts of most of these nutritious foods. The types of food consumed by people of different ethnic, religious, or social backgrounds, as well as different financial statuses, may vary considerably. However, the number of servings of any food depends on its food group as shown in the DASH pyramid.

A balanced plan, such as the DASH diet, includes:

- moderate food consumption and proper calorie intake for body size and physical activity
- an emphasis on plant rather than animal foods
- a variety of foods from different food groups to ensure adequate vitamins and minerals
- keeping a record of the food and calories you consume each day (see Chapter 5)
- increasing one's level of physical activity (see Chapter 7)

Health Benefits of the DASH Diet

The DASH eating plan is extremely beneficial for almost everyone, including those with type 2 diabetes, in whom it can improve the

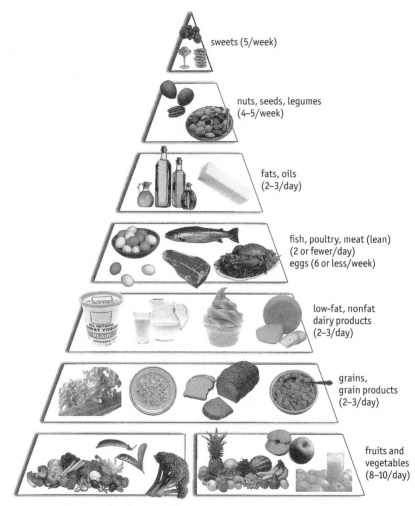

sweets (5/week)

nuts, seeds, legumes
(4–5/week)

fats, oils
(2–3/day)

fish, poultry, meat (lean)
(2 or fewer/day)
eggs (6 or less/week)

low-fat, nonfat
dairy products
(2–3/day)

grains,
grain products
(2–3/day)

fruits and
vegetables
(8–10/day)

FIGURE 15. A proposed DASH pyramid

action of insulin. (See Chapter 8 for more on the DASH diet to treat diabetes.) It promotes vegetables, fruits, and whole grains, and it limits foods high in sugar. The main concern for individuals with type 2 diabetes is the need to consume consistent amounts of food at regular times and in reasonable portion sizes. It is also important for diabetics to control the amount of carbohydrate-containing foods they eat. If you have diabetes, you must consult a physician and a registered dietitian about the exact composition of the foods and beverages you consume.

DASH can also effectively reduce hypertension, risk of stroke, overweight, elevated blood fats, and homocysteine (a substance in the blood that is associated with hardening of the arteries), and it may reduce the risk of kidney stones. In particular, the Omni study (Optimal Macro Nutrient Intake) showed that the beneficial effects of DASH can be enhanced with some adjustments to the plan.[1] Eating less carbohydrate (fruits) and more plant-based protein (legumes, beans), or more monounsaturated fat (olive, canola, safflower oils), further reduced blood fats, slightly decreased blood pressure, and reduced the risk of heart disease.

A special benefit of the DASH eating plan for those who wish to lose weight is that eating lots of fresh vegetables, fresh fruits, whole-grain breads, and whole-grain cereals provides a modest amount of calories with large volumes that may curb the appetite. There is compelling evidence that eating five or more servings of fruits and vegetables a day can reduce the risk of obesity, hypertension, stroke, heart and blood vessel disease, cancer, and type 2 diabetes. In addition to lowering blood pressure, DASH effectively lowers bad cholesterol and reduces the occurrence of stroke.

How effective is the DASH diet in reducing blood pressure? In one study, after eight weeks on DASH, the systolic and diastolic pressures in hypertensive individuals decreased by 11.4 and 5.5 mm Hg, respectively.[2] (Systolic pressure, indicated by the first number in the blood pressure reading, tells how much pressure is being exerted on the walls of the blood vessels when the heart is beating. Diastolic pressure, the second number, indicates how much pressure is being exerted when the heart is between beats, or resting.) These declines exceed those of many studies using drugs. Even persons with high-normal blood pressures experienced a decrease of about 3.5 mm Hg in their diastolic pressure. On the other hand, researchers did not observe any change in blood pressure of individuals consuming typical American diets, which contain approximately 37 percent of calories in the form of fat and are low in fruits and vegetables.

The decrease in blood pressure found with the DASH eating plan occurred without any other lifestyle changes, which indicates the value of decreasing dietary fat and increasing consumption of fruits and vegetables. A second DASH study showed that by further decreasing salt (sodium chloride) consumption, the blood pressure was lowered even more. The lower the salt consumption in the DASH eating plan, the more dramatic the blood pressure–lowering effect.[3]

Studies indicate that increased consumption of potassium is helpful in gradually reducing blood pressure and preventing stroke. Experimental evidence indicates that potassium can dilate blood vessels and thereby lower blood pressure. Furthermore, potassium can maintain a normal circulation in the brain and prevent constriction of blood vessels that can result in strokes, which may occur with excessive salt consumption. Therefore, an eating plan that contains abundant amounts of fruits and vegetables, which are rich in potassium, is particularly healthy. However, in persons with a poorly functioning kidney, dietary potassium may have to be limited, since kidney failure can cause retention of potassium that may be harmful to the heart. There is also evidence that vegetables may play a role in reducing blood pressure by releasing into the blood a chemical called nitric oxide that dilates blood vessels. Because of increased emphasis on fruits, vegetables, nuts, seeds, and legumes (e.g., peas, beans, lentils, soybeans), the potassium content of the DASH diet is roughly two and a half times greater than that of diets ordinarily consumed in the United States. The roles played in decreasing blood pressure by other minerals in fruits and vegetables (such as calcium and magnesium) and by fat reduction are less clear.

Clinically significant short-term weight-loss maintenance was achieved in a diverse population of high-risk patients through moderately intense physical activity combined with the DASH eating plan.[4] However, regaining weight on any diet is extremely common. Therefore, it is uncertain whether DASH will be significantly more successful in combating overweight and obesity and their complications than some of the other popular diets or eating plans. Long-term observations are essential to further evaluate the effectiveness of the DASH eating plan in addressing the obesity crisis.

Choose Foods Wisely: How to Maximize the Benefits of the DASH Plan

The benefits of the foods recommended in the DASH plan are particularly compelling arguments for adhering to the plan whether your weight is in a healthy range or above it. Still, it pays to know which foods recommended by the DASH eating plan confer the most advantageous health effects.

It appears that some salt-responsive hypertensives who are calcium-deficient may lower their blood pressure by consuming foods high in calcium, which may increase excretion of salt and water. Persons with hypertension should be sure to first choose fresh or frozen fruits and vegetables, and then processed foods labeled "low sodium" or "reduced sodium." Those who are lactose intolerant or who otherwise have trouble digesting dairy products can drink lactose-free milk or milk pretreated with lactase enzyme. Also, lactase drops (available at grocery or drug stores) can be added to dairy products, or lactase pills can be taken to prevent indigestion, so that high-calcium dairy foods may still be enjoyed. Calcium-fortified orange juice (and other juices), and soy or rice milk are alternative sources of calcium. Calcium-rich foods can also protect from osteoporosis and possibly colon cancer.

Increasing your consumption of fruits, vegetables, grains, and nuts—all of which contain beneficial chemicals called antioxidants in addition to the crucial vitamins and minerals discussed above—may prevent harmful oxidation of certain chemicals in the body, thereby protecting you from various cancers, hardening of the arteries, heart disease, hypertension, stroke, blood clots, cataracts, and macular degeneration (a cause of blindness). Interestingly, some evidence indicates that children who consume fruits and vegetables daily have healthier arteries in young adulthood than those who eat fruits and vegetables less than twice a month. See Table 4 for a brief list of some antioxidant-rich foods and the protection against disease they may provide, but note that these claims are only suggested, not established. Particularly good sources of antioxidants are fruits (especially berries) and fruit juices, vegetables (especially beans), grains, nuts, herbs, tea, coffee, red wine, and dark chocolate. Whole-grain foods may also protect from cancer, heart disease, stroke, and diabetes. Fruits and vegetables that are deeply colored are particularly rich sources of antioxidants.

Table 4. Beneficial Substances Contained in Some Plant Foods

Food	Substance	Effect on Disease Risk Reduction
Carrots	Antioxidant: beta-carotene	Reduced risk for several types of cancer
Tomatoes	Antioxidant: lycopene	Reduced risk for prostate cancer Reduced risk for heart disease
Grapes/grape juice/ red wine	Phenols, resveratrol	Supports normal, healthy cardio-vascular function
Deep green vegetables	Antioxidant: lutein	May contribute to maintenance of healthy vision and prevention of macular degeneration
Fruit	Anthocyanidins, flavones	May reduce risk of cancer
Cruciferous vegetables (broccoli, kale, cauliflower, collards), horseradish	Sulphoraphane, allyl methyl trisulfide, dithiolethiones	May reduce risk of cancer May lower LDL cholesterol May help to maintain healthy immune system

(cont'd.)

Table 4. Beneficial Substances Contained in Some Plant Foods (cont'd.)

Food	Substance	Effect on Disease Risk Reduction
Blueberries	Antioxidants: phenolic compounds	May lower risk of cancer and heart disease by neutralizing free radicals
Cranberries	Proanthocyanadins	Supports urinary tract health by keeping harmful bacteria from sticking to the walls of the urinary tract

(Source: http://www.dashforhealth.com)

Selecting lean meat and poultry (without the skin) and consuming no more than two servings a day of 3 ounces each (about the size of a deck of cards) will lower the fat and calories you consume.

Fish are an excellent source of protein and contain less saturated fat and cholesterol than beef, pork, or chicken. In addition, many varieties of fish contain omega-3 fatty acid, a polyunsaturated fat recommended for good health. It can lower unhealthy fats (triglycerides) in the blood and can reduce the risk of heart attack, irregular heartbeat, and sudden death. It also may lower blood pressure slightly and prevent dangerous blood clots from forming. Including fish that contain omega-3 fats in your diet—such as fatty cold-water fish, salmon, halibut, tuna, trout, herring, anchovies, sardines, and mackerel—at least two times per week is heart healthy. Even lean cod, flounder, lobster, and crab provide some omega-3 fats. Fish oil supplements can also be beneficial, but consuming large amounts—more than 3 grams of fish oil per day—may increase the risk of bleeding and worsen heart irregularities. Fish oil capsules may contain large doses of vitamin A and D, both of which may be toxic if consumed in megadose amounts. Before taking fish oil supplements, consult your doctor.

It is noteworthy that Eskimos, who consume a large amount of fish, have relatively low levels of cholesterol and triglycerides in their blood and rarely have heart disease. As mentioned previously, persons should limit consumption of swordfish, shark, tile, mackerel, and albacore tuna to once a week or less often, since these fish may contain significant amounts of mercury. Women who are pregnant or trying to become pregnant, nursing mothers, and children under five years old should limit the amount of fish they eat and should avoid fish that may contain mercury.

Whole grains should take the place of foods made with refined flour (such as white-flour breads, bagels, crackers, and rolls). Sugar and foods high in sugar (e.g., candy, cake, ice cream, pastries, cookies, and other baked goods) can be eaten occasionally. Choose fruit butters that do not have added sugar. Nuts provide protein and healthy types of fat, but they are high in calories and should be eaten only in recommended amounts. As discussed in some detail earlier in the chapter, avoid foods high in saturated fats and trans fats. Monounsaturated fats (e.g., olive or canola oil, or omega-3 fats in fish) are particularly healthful, but like other fats they are high in calories, so stick with the recommended amounts. If you want a spread for your breakfast toast (whole-grain, of course), a fat-free alternative is to choose a "fruit butter" such as apple butter, which does not actually contain butter but is a fruit spread.

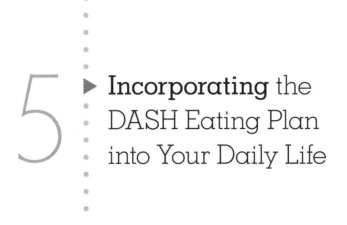

5 ▶ Incorporating the DASH Eating Plan into Your Daily Life

▶ Adopting a healthy eating plan involves more than just finding the right diet. There are some beneficial strategies to follow—both behavioral and mental. This chapter offers practical advice for *how* to integrate the DASH diet (or, really, any nutritious eating plan) into your everyday life.

Good Strategies for Healthy Eating

Let us start with a general list of pointers for healthy eating. These are strategies that everyone can benefit from—whether their goal is to maintain an ideal weight or to lose weight.

- **Use a smaller plate** when eating so that you put less food on your plate. The obesity rate in Italy and France is reported to be 70 percent lower than in the United States. It has been suggested that one reason may be the use in those countries of a ten-inch-diameter food plate instead of the twelve-inch plate used in the United States. Of course, the caloric content and amount of the food determines its effect on body weight.

- **Avoid second helpings.** Just say no!
- **When dining out, eat only a portion of the meal.** Take the remainder home for a meal at another time, or leave it at the restaurant.
- **Avoid frying.** Instead, bake, broil, steam, grill, boil, sauté (in broth, olive oil, or nonstick spray), poach, or roast.
- **Reduce consumption of calorie-dense foods containing added sugar and solid fat.**
- **Choose low-fat or no-fat dairy products.**
- **Eat more slowly.** Doing so will cause you to feel fuller.
- **Drink a glass of water or fat-free milk about fifteen minutes before eating a meal to help curb your appetite. Consuming low-calorie soups with meals will also help make you feel full.** However, most soups contain lots of salt, and anyone trying to reduce consumption of sodium may have to limit soups or should choose reduced-sodium soups, which are now available.
- **Reduce consumption of sodas and juices with added sugars.** Diet sodas are permissible, but another reason to limit sodas is to avoid excess caffeine consumption.
- **Divide your plate into three sections: ¼ for starch (grains), ¼ for fish, poultry, or lean meat, and ½ for vegetables and/or fruits.** By doing this, you can control portion sizes and avoid overeating (see Figure 16).

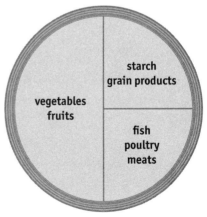

FIGURE 16. Your dinner plate

- **If you snack between meals, choose healthful snacks** such as the following: 1 fresh fruit, ½ cup cut vegetables with salsa, 3 cups unsalted popcorn (air popped with no fat added, or low-fat microwave popcorn), 2 rice cakes, 4 slices melba toast, 3 graham crackers, 1 cup of low-fat yogurt, or diet gelatin. Avoid calorie-dense foods and sugary drinks at the movies and at home while watching TV.

- **Increase consumption of fruits** at breakfast and in place of high-calorie desserts.

- **Learn which foods to choose and which to limit from each food group** (see Table 5).

Table 5. Foods to Choose vs. Foods to Limit: An Excellent Guide to Healthy Eating

Food Groups	Foods to Choose	Foods to Limit
Grains, Starches	Whole-grain breads and hot or cold cereals (with little or no added sugar), rice cakes, whole-grain crackers, pasta, brown rice, corn, sweet and white potatoes	Doughnuts, pastries, croissants, biscuits, refined muffins, sugary cereals, French toast, crackers made with fat, granola-type cereals, stuffing, fried potatoes, fried rice, French fries
Fruits and Vegetables	Fresh, frozen, or canned fruits, fresh or frozen vegetables, dried fruits, fruit and vegetable juices (check labels to make sure none have added sugar or salt)	Coconut, fried vegetables, prepared or packaged foods in cream, butter, oil, cheese sauce
Dairy Products	Skim milk, 1 percent or fat-free milk, skim buttermilk, nonfat and low-fat yogurt and cottage cheese, low-fat cheeses (containing no more than 3 g of fat per serving)	2 percent and whole milk, buttermilk, cream, butter, half and half, cheeses made from whole milk and cream, whole-milk cottage cheese, cream cheese, whole-milk ricotta, mozzarella, or imitation hard cheeses, sour cream, heavy and whipping cream, regular yogurt

(cont'd.)

Table 5. Foods to Choose vs. Foods to Limit: An Excellent Guide to Healthy Eating (cont'd.)

Food Groups	Foods to Choose	Foods to Limit
Fish, Poultry, Meat, Eggs	Fish, shellfish, tuna packed in water, chicken and turkey without skin, lean cuts of beef, lamb, veal, or pork, venison, egg yolks (limit to six or fewer per week), egg substitute, egg whites	Prime-grade fatty cuts of beef, lamb, or pork, fast-food hamburgers, ribs, bacon, sausage, duck, goose, regular cold cuts, hot dogs, tuna packed in oil, organ meats, ham hocks, fast-food chicken nuggets
Nuts, Seeds, Legumes	Unsalted nuts and seeds, dry or canned (low-sodium) lentils, beans, black beans, and peas, soybeans, peanut butter	Prepared canned beans and lentils, salted nuts and seeds
Fats & Oils	Vegetable oils (1 tsp), margarine (1 tsp), diet margarine (1 Tbsp); mayonnaise: regular (1 tsp), reduced-fat (1 Tbsp); salad dressing: regular (1 Tbsp), low-fat (2 Tbsp)	Coconut or palm oil (mostly found in baked goods), butter, whipped butter, shortening or lard, high-calorie salad dressings (e.g., containing cheese)
Seasonings, Sweets, Miscellaneous	All herbs and spices (without salt), pepper, mustard, low-sodium ketchup, vinegar, hot sauce, lemon or lime juice, low-sodium soy sauce, sorbet, nonfat ice cream and frozen yogurt, flavored ices, angel food cake, fig bars, graham crackers, meringues, pudding made with skim milk, cocoa powder, plain popcorn, hard candy, jelly beans, maple syrup, jelly, jams, gelatin	Barbecue sauce, cream sauces, cheese sauces, cakes, cookies, pies, pastries, ice cream, chocolate, regular pudding, milkshakes, buttered popcorn, potato chips and other fried snacks such as corn chips or tortilla chips, pickles, salted pretzels

Tips for Losing Weight

If your goal is weight reduction, once you've found a good eating plan you need to think about what else is involved in losing weight. That's the focus of this section.

1. Remember that losing excess weight requires, above all, determination and persistence in pursuing a healthy lifestyle. For this reason, make changes slowly. In addition, some may find it especially helpful to lose weight with a friend or a group of individuals who also are trying to lose weight. Overeaters Anonymous encourages groups of overweight individuals to work together to lose weight mainly by reducing the amount of calories they eat. The group programs Weight Watchers and Jenny Craig incorporate healthy eating plans and emphasize increased physical activity. Many find a group approach very helpful and are able to lose weight and keep it off for as long as they stick with the program.

2. Be aware that there are no magic diets or pills. There are all sorts of special diets that often make fraudulent and unscientific claims of dramatically reducing weight. However, the fact that 95 percent of persons who lose weight eventually regain it indicates that short-term diets are not the answer. The key is to make life-long changes that result in *both* choosing healthful foods in moderation *and* becoming more physically active. So-called "crash" or "fad" diets that produce very rapid weight loss by severely restricting calories can be dangerous for some people. In particular, high-fat diets may be harmful to patients with high blood cholesterol levels, atherosclerosis (hardening of the arteries), diabetes, or poor kidney or liver function. Chapter 6 offers a quick rundown of several popular weight-loss programs.

One of the shortcomings of most weight-loss diets, except the DASH eating plan and the Pritikin diet, a very low-fat diet that was popular in the 1980s (see Chapter 6), is that none of them mention or stress the importance of limiting the use of salt. As previously discussed, salt limitation is very important in the prevention and treatment of hypertension, and it should be recommended in almost every diet. In addition to its food recommendations, the DASH eating plan emphasizes the importance of limiting salt consumption. More recently, the principles of the DASH plan have been incorporated into the Mayo Clinic Healthy-Weight Pyramid.

The federal government, the National Academy of Sciences, and the Center for Science in the Public Interest all recommend that Americans reduce their salt consumption. See Chapter 9 for more on the importance of limiting salt intake.

With any special diet, particularly when the goal is weight reduction, it is important to make certain that the diet is nutritionally adequate and that vitamin and mineral deficiencies are avoided. These deficiencies are important to recognize and remedy, particularly for those who reduce food consumption to lose weight. With vegetarian diets, which are usually low in fat and very healthy, care must be taken to ensure adequate intake of fortified foods (such as cereals that have added iron and vitamin B_{12}) and, for vegans (those who avoid eating all animal foods, including eggs and dairy products), foods containing nonanimal calcium. Dietary supplements of vitamins, calcium, and iron may be needed for some vegetarians and for others on a weight-reduction diet, particularly when calories are limited to 1,200 or fewer daily.

Comments by Dr. T. Colin Campbell (Professor Emeritus of Nutritional Biochemistry at Cornell University) are particularly pertinent to diet and weight loss. He points out that consuming diets high in animal protein and fat tends to increase body fat and weight gain. Furthermore, for the most effective weight-loss plan, he emphasizes the importance of consuming fresh fruits and vegetables and whole-grain foods, plus a reasonable amount of exercise. He indicates that fat intake increases with animal-protein consumption, and that saturated fat and cholesterol are responsible for increasing the concentration of bad (LDL) blood cholesterol. In their book, *The China Study,* Dr. Campbell and his son, Dr. Thomas M. Campbell II, reported that death from coronary artery heart disease was seventeen times higher among Americans than rural Chinese.

Dr. Campbell emphasizes that avoidance of animal-based foods and increased consumption of plant-based proteins and fats, and fresh fruits and vegetables, is an especially healthy diet; however, he notes that unfortunately many persons attempting to lose weight become "junk-food vegetarians" by replacing meat with dairy foods, oils, refined carbohydrates, pastas made with refined grains, sweets, and pastries. These foods are non-nutritious and often cause weight gain instead of weight loss.

As recently pointed out by the Mayo Clinic, strict vegetarian diets that prohibit animal fats—or those that permit some animal products such as eggs and dairy—can reduce weight since they are more filling and less calorie dense. However, weight gain on a vegetarian diet can occur if you eat very large portions of fruits and vegetables or consume high-calorie foods such as sugar-sweetened beverages, desserts, snack foods, soy hot dogs, soy cheeses, or refried beans. The Mayo Clinic recommends that vegetarians eat a variety of fruits and vegetables, whole or enriched grains, legumes, seeds, nuts, and low-fat dairy products. It can also be helpful to limit foods and beverages that are highly sweetened, as well as high-fat foods such as nuts, oils, sour cream, mayonnaise, and salad dressing—or to use their low-fat versions.

Recent reliable reports confirm that "no particular combination of protein, carbohydrate, and fat in the diet offers any advantage in losing weight."[1] Yet, on the other hand, some experts believe that certain people lose weight—and maintain weight loss—more successfully on an eating plan that limits one or more of the macronutrients (carbohydrate, protein, or fat). If that is indeed true, recent studies suggest that a simple genetic test may determine whether an individual should consume a low-fat or a low-carbohydrate diet to lose weight. These results are preliminary, but, if confirmed, such a test may prove valuable in diet selection.

For now, most experts still agree that weight loss depends on reduced calorie consumption and increased calorie burning rather than on a particular diet composition. To lose excess weight, you must eat fewer calories than what you have been consuming, and you should burn more calories through physical activity. It is important to stress that weight loss can be easier with *healthy* food consumption and adequate exercise. Exercise also increases lean body mass (muscle tissue), which will increase your metabolism, thereby causing your body to burn more calories. Chapter 7 goes into some detail about the exercise part of the formula.

Reduction of saturated fat, carbohydrate (especially sugar), and portion size is key. It is important to recognize that processed foods labeled "low fat" or "no fat" may have as many or more calories than the regular fat-containing food item. You should always read food labels. Finally, it is most helpful to follow a weight-loss program that offers support services (a registered dietitian, an exercise therapist, and other experts) to guide and encourage your efforts and to monitor your food consumption and weight loss.

3. Consider eating a large volume of food if it is low in calories; this will help you feel full and will curb your appetite. A recently proposed "volumetric" diet to lose weight is based on this strategy. For the same reason, do not skip meals. Skipping meals will not reduce weight but can increase BMI, since excess calories are often eaten at other meals. In particular, it is important to heed the advice given in the next tip.

4. Eat breakfast. Especially if you are trying to lose weight. It may seem reasonable to skip breakfast in the belief that you will thereby reduce daily calories consumed. However, skipping breakfast can markedly increase your appetite for lunch, resulting in the consumption of many more calories at lunch and thus increasing your total caloric intake. Furthermore, strong evidence proves that skipping breakfast can reduce concentration and performance—especially in schoolwork.

Breakfast is a great opportunity to increase your fiber intake in the form of grain cereal, bread, and fruit. Adequate fiber will curb appetite and help reduce weight. It is reported that doubling your fiber consumption can cause a weight loss of ten pounds per year.

5. Weigh yourself once a week, and be patient. A slow, gradual weight loss of one to two pounds weekly adds up to a significant loss over time. Do not be discouraged if you lose more weight in one week and less in another. Permanent weight loss is not a race. Slow and steady wins the game. Many studies show that rapid weight loss is typically followed by regaining lost weight.

6. Have a sense of your daily caloric needs, and learn how your food choices can meet—or exceed—those needs. The calories your body burns each day depend on your weight, level of physical activity, and muscular composition. Those with more muscle mass burn more calories. The DASH eating plan outlined in Table 3 of the last chapter is equivalent to about 2,000 calories. To maintain a healthy weight, most American women need about 1,600 calories per day, and most American men need about 2,200. Of course, the very physically active will require more calories (e.g., about 2,200 for women, and about 2,800 for men). Normally active teenage males may require up to 2,800 calories—much more if they're very physically active. Normally active teenage females need about 2,200 calories, or more if they're very physically active.

If you are interested in estimating the number of daily calories you need to maintain an ideal weight, a simple calculation follows. First, determine the ideal body weight (IBW) for your height and frame size by reviewing Table 1 on page 16. Then:

- Multiply IBW by 13 if you are **sedentary** (performing little if any exercise). For example, a sedentary person with an ideal weight of 150 pounds requires 1,950 calories (i.e., 13 × 150 = 1,950).

- Multiply IBW by 15 if you are **moderately active** (exercising four to five times a week). For example, a moderately active person with an ideal weight of 150 pounds requires 2,250 calories (i.e., 15 × 150 = 2,250).

- Multiply IBW by 17 if you are **very active** (training or exercising ten or more hours a week). For example, a very active person with an ideal weight of 150 pounds requires 2,550 calories (i.e., 17 × 150 = 2,550).

Table 6 gives a more-detailed estimate of the daily calorie requirement for women and men based on weight and level of physical activity.

Table 6. How Many Calories You Need Each Day

Weight (pounds)	Less Active	Moderately Active	Very Active	Weight (pounds)	Less Active	Moderately Active	Very Active
Women				**Men**			
100	1,178	1,473	1,669	120	1,571	1,964	2,225
110	1,296	1,620	1,836	130	1,702	2,127	2,411
120	1,414	1,767	2,003	140	1,833	2,291	2,596
130	1,532	1,915	2,170	150	1,964	2,455	2,782
140	1,649	2,062	2,337	160	2,095	2,618	2,967
150	1,767	2,209	2,504	170	2,225	2,782	3,153
160	1,885	2,356	2,671	180	2,356	2,945	3,338
170	2,003	2,504	2,837	190	2,487	3,109	3,524
180	2,121	2,651	3,004	200	2,618	3,273	3,709
190	2,239	2,798	3,171	210	2,749	3,436	3,895
200	2,356	2,945	3,338	220	2,880	3,600	4,080
210	2,474	3,093	3,505	230	3,011	3,764	4,265
220	2,592	3,240	3,672	240	3,142	3,927	4,451
230	2,710	3,387	3,839	250	3,273	4,091	4,636
240	2,828	3,535	4,006	260	3,404	4,255	4,822
250	2,945	3,682	4,173	270	3,535	4,418	5,007

(Source: *The Dash Diet for Hypertension,* with permission.)

How many calories should you consume if you're trying to lose weight? To lose about one pound a week, a simple rule of thumb is to multiply ten times your current weight in pounds, or multiply twenty-two times your current weight in kilograms. For example, if you weigh 150 pounds, you will lose about a pound a week if you consume about 1,500 calories per day.

Another way of thinking about it is to know that reducing food and beverage consumption by 500 calories per day usually results in weight loss of about one pound per week. This is most easily done by decreasing the size and number of servings you eat (see Tables 3 and 7) and increasing your level of physical activity. By closely following the recommended number of servings, you will reduce your intake of fat, sugar, sweets, and snacks. As already emphasized, you should never skip meals, since this may result in consuming excessive calories at the next meal. And breakfast is an important meal because it supplies energy to efficiently perform mental and physical activities in the morning, and it curbs the appetite for lunch.

In general, diets containing 1,000–1,200 calories per day for women and 1,200–1,600 calories per day for men will usually produce a steady and safe rate of weight loss (one to two pounds per week), especially if combined with exercise. Very-low-calorie diets (fewer than 800 calories per day) are not recommended without physician supervision.

Table 7 indicates the calories contained in one serving of food in the various food groups. Table 8 on page 87 indicates the approximate calorie requirement and servings of each food group for children, teenagers, and adults, as recommended by the U.S. Department of Agriculture (the number of servings depends on age). However, the DASH eating plan emphasizes daily consumption of four to five servings *each* of fruits and vegetables for adults; that is, approximately eight to ten total servings per day of fruits and vegetables. In one DASH study, participants following the plan never felt hungry.[2]

Table 7. Food Groups, Examples, and Calorie Content

Food	Serving size*
Fruits: about 60 calories/serving	
Fresh fruit	1 small piece
Berries	¾ to 1 C**
Canned, packed in water or fruit juice	½ C
Dried fruit	2 Tbsp
Nonstarchy Vegetables: about 50 calories/serving	
Raw	2 C
Cooked vegetables or vegetable juice	1 C
Grains: about 80 calories/serving (whole grains are recommended, including cereals, grains, pasta, breads, crackers, and starchy vegetables)	
Rice or pasta	⅓ C
Cooked or dry cereal, starchy vegetable	½ C
Breads (small roll, ½ English muffin, 6-inch tortilla)	1 slice or 1 item
Crackers, unsalted pretzels	¾ to 1 oz (check label for number of pieces)
Low-fat, Nonfat Dairy Products: about 90 to 120 calories/serving unless otherwise specified	
Skim, 1 percent, or 2 percent milk	1 C
Fat-free, low-fat buttermilk	1 C
Nonfat or low-fat yogurt, plain or fruit flavored and artificially sweetened	⅔ C
Cheese:	
1 gram fat or less/ounce (35 calories)	1 oz
3 grams fat or less/ounce (55 calories)	1 oz
Cottage cheese:	
nonfat or low-fat (35 calories)	¼ C
4.5 grams fat or less/ounce (55 calories)	¼ C
Lean Meats, Poultry, Fish: lean meats have about 45 calories (≤ 3 g fat) per serving; medium-fat meats have about 75 calories (≤ 5 g fat) per serving	
Beef, pork, lamb, veal, game	1 oz cooked
Poultry (remove skin)	1 oz cooked
Fish (fresh, frozen, canned–water pack)	1 oz cooked
Shellfish (clams, crab, lobster, scallops, shrimp)	1 oz cooked
Eggs:	
Whole–limit to 6 or fewer/week	1
Egg whites	3
Egg substitute	¼ C

(cont'd.)

Table 7. Food Groups, Examples, and Calorie Content (cont'd.)

Food	Serving size*
Fats and Oils: about 45 calories/serving:	
Margarine (trans-fat free):	
Stick, tub, or squeeze	1 tsp
Low-fat	1 Tbsp
Mayonnaise:	
Regular	1 tsp
Reduced-fat	1 Tbsp
Salad dressing:	
Regular	1 tsp
Reduced-fat	2 Tbsp
Vegetable oils (olive, corn, safflower, sunflower, etc.)	1 tsp
Nuts, Seeds, Legumes (Beans, Peas, Lentils, Soy Products): Calories—specified according to category	
Nuts **(about 90 calories)**	
Almonds, cashews, mixed	12 nuts
Peanuts	20 nuts
Pecans, walnuts	8 halves
Nut and seed spreads **(about 180 calories)**	
Peanut butter, almond butter, tahini	2 Tbsp
Seeds **(about 80 calories)**	
Sunflower or pumpkin seed kernels	2 Tbsp
Tofu **(about 190 calories)**	
Firm, regular	1 C
Firm, light	2 C
Legumes, cooked (about 115 calories) **	
Split peas, lentils**	½ C
Beans (black, garbanzo, kidney, lima, navy, pinto, white)**	½ C
Beans, baked**	⅓ C
** Need to also count as carbohydrate serving	
Sweets (About 100 calories/serving)	
Candy bar (milk chocolate)	½ of 1.5 oz bar
M&Ms (plain)	½ of 1.6 oz package
Jelly beans or Lifesavers	10 each

* Number of daily servings will depend on daily calorie consumption
** C = cup
(Source: Adapted from the U.S. Department of Agriculture)

Table 8. How Many Servings Do You Need Each Day?

(Recommended by the U.S. Department of Agriculture for children, teens, and adults)

Food group	Children ages 2 to 6 years, women, some older adults (about 1,600 calories) Servings	Older children, teen girls, active women, most men (about 2,200 calories) Servings	Teen boys, active men (about 2,800 calories) Servings
Grains Group (bread, cereal, rice, and pasta, especially whole grain)	6	9	11
Vegetable group	3	4	5
Fruit Group	2	3	4
Milk Group (milk, yogurt, and cheese—preferably fat-free or low-fat)	2 or 3*	2 or 3*	2 or 3*
Meat and Beans Group (meat, poultry, fish, dry beans, eggs, and nuts—preferably lean or low fat)	2, for a total of 5 oz	2, for a total of 6 oz	3, for a total of 7 oz

(Adapted from U.S. Department of Agriculture, Center for Nutrition Policy and Promotion, with modifications)
* The number of servings depends on your age. Older children and teenagers (ages 9 to 18 years) and adults over the age of 50 need 3 servings daily. Others need 2 servings daily. During pregnancy and lactation, the recommended number of milk-group servings is the same as that of nonpregnant women.

It is important to read food and beverage labels and become aware of their macronutrient, fiber, salt, and calorie content. However, most important of all is simply to learn the serving sizes and number of daily servings from each food group that you should consume for your calorie requirement (see Tables 3 and 9. Table 9 on the next page shows the number of daily servings recommended by the DASH eating plan for each caloric range).

7. Recognize the dangers of snacking. Individuals who gain weight or become obese often do so partly because they select high-calorie, non-nutritious foods and snacks, and they "supersize" their portions. Keep snack portions small. Donuts, pastries, most muffins,

Table 9. How Many Servings You Need Each Day from Each Food Group for Various Calorie Requirements (DASH Eating Plan)

Calorie-intake range	Grains	Vege-tables	Fruits	Dairy foods	Meats, poultry, and fish	Nuts, seeds, and legumes	Added fats and oils	Sweets
1,400–1800	6	4	4	2	1½	¼	1	½
1,800–2,200	7	4	4	2½	1½	½	2	½
2,200–2,600	9	5	5	3	2	½	3	1
2,600–3,000	11	6	6	3½	2½	½	4	2

(Source: *The Dash Diet For Hypertension,* with permission)

cakes, crackers, cookies, chips, and all sorts of candies and sweets are high in fat, sugar, and calories. These snacks do not have to be totally eliminated, but they should usually be replaced with fruits and vegetables. Raw fruit, celery and carrot sticks, broccoli, cauliflower, unbuttered and unsalted popcorn, unsalted whole-wheat pretzels, graham crackers, low-fat or fat-free yogurt, and snack crackers (e.g., Finn Crisps, matzoh, etc.) contain little or no fat, relatively few calories, and may effectively relieve hunger.

The calories contained in several popular snack foods are listed in Table 10.

Table 10. Calorie and Fat Content of Popular Snack Foods

Snack Type	Calories	Fat (g)
Apple, medium (3 in diameter)	95	0
Banana, small (6 to 7 in long)	90	0
Cantaloupe (¼ medium melon)	46	0
Carrots (4 oz)	22	0
Chips (1 bag)	150–500	10–33
Donut	165–300	8–20

(cont'd.)

Table 10. Calorie and Fat Content of Popular Snack Foods (cont'd.)

Snack Type	Calories	Fat (g)
Danish pastry (2.5 oz)	220–280	6–12
Fat-free frozen yogurt (½ C*)	100	0
Fat-free granola bar	95	1
Granola bar	100–260	4–10
Grapefruit half (about 4 in diameter)	55	0
Low-fat frozen yogurt (½ C)	145	4
M&M (1 regular-size bag)	236	10
Orange, medium	50	0
Orange, small (about 2½ in diameter)	45	0
Peach, medium (about 1 C of slices)	60	0
Pear, small (about 1 C of slices)	86	0
Popcorn (1 C) air popped white cheddar sour cream and chive	31 55 50	0 3 3
Pretzels (1 oz)	108–120	1
Snickers bar	273	14

* C = cup
(Source: dashforhealth.com, with slight modifications)

Choose high-fiber snacks—for example, vegetables, fruits, whole-grain foods (e.g., whole-grain breads and cereals, whole-wheat pasta, brown rice, barley, legumes, nuts, and whole-wheat, low-fat snack crackers, etc.). Because it is higher in bulk, dietary fiber is filling and curbs the appetite; it has been found to be effective in cutting calories and controlling weight. It also promotes regular bowel function. And, as previously mentioned, there is convincing evidence that consumption of dietary fiber lowers cholesterol absorption from the intestine.

Whole-grain foods are healthier than processed grains (e.g., white bread and white rice) because they maintain their natural

nutrients and fiber. Nuts contain healthy fats that can lower cholesterol and reduce the risk of heart attacks. They are a great substitute
for unhealthy snacks; however, for those trying to lose weight, nuts
must be limited to avoid excess consumption of fat calories.

The healthiest snacks are fresh fruits and vegetables because
they are low in calories and high in nutrition; they have lots of vitamins, minerals, antioxidants (protective chemicals), and fiber. Fruit
and vegetable juices are very nutritious; however, they do not provide nearly the amount of fiber present in fresh fruits and veggies.
Many vegetable juices, such as V8, also contain a very high sodium
content, which is undesirable. Low-sodium V8 and vegetable juices
are preferable to regular versions. Fruit juices are low in sodium
and high in potassium, which is beneficial because, as already mentioned, potassium can lower elevated blood pressure and reduce
the risk of a stroke.

Some high-fiber foods and their calorie content are listed in
Table 11.

Table 11. High-Fiber Foods and Their Calorie Content

Food	Calories	Fiber (g)
All Bran, ½ C*	75	13
Apple, 1 medium	94	4
Chickpeas, ½ C	134	6
Cooked carrots	27	2
Corn, ½ C	89	2
Green peas, ½ C	67	4
Kidney beans, ½ C	112	11
Pears, 1 medium	95	4
Raisin Bran, 1 C	190	6.5
Raspberries, ½ C	32	4

* C = cup
(Source: dashforhealth.com, with modification)

8. Drink lots of fluids to help control the urge to snack. Aim for six to eight glasses daily of water or other low-calorie drinks. Water is calorie free and a great stand-in for other calorie-free beverages when you are thirsty. Although milk and fruit juice are healthful, they do contribute easy-to-consume calories. Whole milk should be replaced with fat-free (skim) or low-fat milk. Fruit juice should be 100 percent unsweetened and limited to 8 ounces per day, and soda and drinks containing sugar should be avoided and replaced with sugarless "diet" drinks or calorie-free flavored sparkling water. For your tea and coffee, use noncaloric sweeteners or very little sugar, and fat-free or low-fat milk.

9. But don't overdo it on the caffeine-containing beverages. Most adults are aware that excess caffeine consumption can cause nervousness, irritability, anxiety, shakiness, insomnia, and an inability to relax and concentrate. It also may produce a temporary increase in heart rate and blood pressure and sometimes an irregular heart beat in persons who are hypertensive or normotensive (have normal blood pressure). The content of caffeine is greater in coffee than in tea or soft drinks; it is even lower in cocoa and chocolate products. Therefore, it is best for most persons (particularly those with hypertension) to consume no more than two cups of coffee, four cups of tea, *or* (not *and*) four cans of caffeinated diet sodas daily. Caffeine in sodas may cause insomnia in children. One benefit of drinking tea rather than other caffeinated or even decaffeinated beverages is that it contains healthful antioxidants. Learn to read the labels on bottles or cans to determine a beverage's sugar and calorie content and whether it contains caffeine. There should be very few sweets or high-calorie snacks or sugary drinks available in the house. Chocolate contains a small amount of caffeine and should be limited in very young children.

10. About fifteen minutes before a meal, to curb your appetite and reduce the calories you consume at the meal, eat a serving

of raw fruits or vegetables, or drink a nutritious low-calorie beverage (e.g., fat-free milk, low-sodium V8 juice). Or start your meal with an appetizer of low-calorie soup. Practically all canned soups and those prepared in restaurants have a high salt content to improve flavor. Gazpacho (chilled tomato soup), however, can be prepared with herbs and spices and with relatively little salt. Take advantage of the low-sodium soups that are available. Eating a large salad with olive oil and vinegar dressing as your main course at lunch or before your main course at dinner provides nutrition as well as a sense of fullness. And it bears repeating that eating slowly and paying attention to what you eat may make you feel fuller so that you eat less. Avoid eating if you are not hungry. We tend to eat too much too fast!

11. If you consume alcohol, avoid drinking more than one drink (for women) or two drinks (for men) per day. This is essential not only to limit calories (1 gram of alcohol contains 7 calories), but also because moderate and excess consumption of alcohol can cause hypertension and may cause stroke. Remember that some alcoholic drinks, especially those containing added mixers, afford lots of calories without any nutritional value. Furthermore, of considerable concern is a recent report in the *Journal of the National Cancer Institute* indicating that even one drink daily may increase the risk of breast, rectal, and liver cancer.[3]

12. Be aware that if you stop smoking, you may tend to gain weight. This occurs because the body's metabolic rate (the rate at which it burns up the calories in food) decreases. The weight gain triggered by quitting smoking can be easily offset by an increase in physical activity—otherwise it will require a further reduction in calories consumed.

13. Consider using a pedometer to record your physical activity. Most adults take two thousand to five thousand steps daily.

It has been recommended that adults take ten thousand or more steps each day to maintain adequate physical activity. The distance traveled depends, of course, on the stride of the individual, that is, the distance in feet made with each step. The average step taken by adults is about 2.5 feet; therefore, ten thousand steps is equivalent to about 4.73 miles. Charts supplied with most pedometers can help you convert stride length and steps taken to miles walked. Although children, adolescents, and teenagers may walk or run this distance daily, most adults do not have the motivation and will not find the time to exercise regularly. Children, adolescents, and teenagers should be physically active for one or more hours daily, whereas to maintain physical fitness, adults should exercise at least thirty minutes five or more days each week.

Walking is very healthy, can be done by almost everyone, and requires no special skills, equipment, or conditioning. It is providential that over two thousand years ago, Hippocrates, the father of medicine, said that "walking is man's best medicine." Obesity is relatively uncommon in societies throughout the world where individuals remain very active physically. Even in the United States, very few Amish, who are reported to be about six times as active as most Americans, become obese, despite a diet "heavy in meat, eggs, bread, and pies."[4] Exercise tends to decrease appetite.[5] Review Chapter 7 for more on the importance of exercise, and keep an accurate record of the amount of exercise you perform daily.

14. If you're tempted to use diet drugs, prescription or nonprescription, only do so under the supervision of a physician. We touched on the topic of nonprescription weight-loss supplements in Chapter 3. In addition to those unregulated (and potentially dangerous) drugs, some prescription drugs have been developed for weight loss. The most popular is orlistat (trade name Xenical), which decreases digestion and absorption of some fats from the intestine. It inhibits about 30 percent of fat absorption, but since it prevents absorption of some fat-soluble vitamins (A, D, E, and beta-carotene), these must be replaced by taking vitamin pills two hours before or two hours after taking orlistat. The drug may cause some diarrhea, bloating, and abdominal pain.

15. Keep a record of your weight and of the food you eat each day. A daily food diary can be extremely helpful; it should include both the foods you eat *and* the amounts consumed. Such record keeping will alert you to excess calorie consumption.

16. Get seven to nine hours of sleep daily. Obtaining adequate sleep appears to decrease the risk of obesity. It has recently been reported that persons sleeping only six, five, or two to four hours were 23 percent, 50 percent, and 73 percent, respectively, more likely to be obese than those getting seven to nine hours sleep. Shorter amounts of sleep cause an increase in a circulating hormone, ghrelin, that stimulates appetite, and a decrease in another circulating hormone, leptin, that ordinarily suppresses appetite. Those hormonal changes are then responsible for excess food consumption and weight gain.

17. If you're morbidly obese (more than one hundred pounds overweight) and unable to lose weight, learn about the pros and cons of undergoing bariatric surgery. As discussed in Chapter 3, bariatric surgery can very effectively reduce weight and cause remission of type 2 diabetes. But the procedure is very serious and has numerous potential complications. If you're considering weight-loss surgery, talk to more than one doctor about the benefits and drawbacks of the various procedures.

18. Shop smart. Only shop for foods when you are not hungry, make a list of what you need, and stick to it. Following this advice means you will be less apt to buy unnecessary items that only add calories to be consumed later by you and your family members. You will also save money by buying less. When you do shop for groceries, it is especially important to include foods recommended in the DASH eating plan. Finally, you should periodically shop for food with your children to familiarize them with healthful foods and to educate them about the importance of limiting fast foods and convenience foods that contain excess fat, sugar, and salt. Permitting children to take part in making healthy choices can influence the food they consume and their future health. Your actions can set a wonderful example that impacts you and your entire family. The importance of example was powerfully expressed by C. S. Lewis: "What you do screams so loudly that I cannot hear what you say."

DASH Guidance for Shopping

That last pointer ("shop smart") is so important we decided to devote an entire section to it. The following guidelines mostly apply when you're shopping for processed foods. Few of us need to rein in our cravings when selecting fresh, unprocessed fruits and vegetables. Feel free to load your grocery cart with those nutrient-packed items. But inevitably you'll also need to include some processed foods in your meal planning. These pointers, which are taken from www.dashforhealth.com, can help you make good choices.

- First, know—and adopt—the **three cardinal rules of grocery shopping** (these bear repeating):
  1. Never go shopping if you are hungry.
  2. Make a list of the foods you really need and then stick to the list.
  3. Learn to read labels and determine the calories and nutritional content of one serving.
- **Fresh foods** are usually found on the perimeter of supermarkets, and processed foods are usually located on the inner aisles. Do most of your shopping on the perimeters.
- **Canned fruits and vegetables** that are packed in liquids

containing sugar and salt are always higher in calories and sodium than fresh fruits and vegetables. **Frozen fruits and vegetables** are a better choice than canned because they usually do not have added sugar, and many contain no added salt. Select those in boxes or bags that do not have sauces that contain calories and sodium. Look for 100 percent pure frozen or canned juices, and avoid fruit-flavored drinks and punches, which have added sugar. Look for fruit packaged without sugar.

- **Beans and peas (fresh or dried)** are an inexpensive source of protein and contain healthy fiber, folic acid, iron, and minerals. If desired, canned beans can be rinsed with water for several minutes to reduce the sodium content (salt is usually added during canning to expedite the process; today, no-salt canned beans and tomatoes are also available in many stores).

- **Whole grain and yolk-free pastas and brown rice** are good sources of complex carbohydrates.

- **Tomato-based sauces, or herbs and olive oil,** can be used in place of creamed sauces and butter. This will enhance flavor and reduce the need for salt. Try making your own pasta sauces, and keep added salt to a minimum.

- Read the labels of **canned soups,** since they usually have a very high sodium content. However, some low-sodium soups are acceptable, especially if seasoned with herbs and spices to improve flavor. Better yet, make your own. Cream-based soups can add significant calories and should be avoided by those trying to lose weight. Use fat-free milk or water to reconstitute condensed soups, instead of whole milk or cream.

- When choosing **salad dressings or mayonnaise, or mayonnaise-type dressings,** use low-calorie, low-fat, or fat-free versions. If you use a regular dressing, you can decrease fat and calories by adding water, fat-free milk, or plain, low, or nonfat yogurt.

- Most **vegetable oils** are made from healthy unsaturated fats. The healthiest vegetable oils contain monounsaturated fat (e.g., olive, canola, peanut, and avocado oils). Olive oil has the highest content of monounsaturated fat and is especially beneficial for heart health. Polyunsaturated fats (contained in safflower, sunflower, corn, and soybean oils) are also healthy. No matter the type, however, oils are high in calories and should be limited if weight reduction is desired. Vegetable cooking sprays will keep the use of cooking oil to a minimum.

- **Hot and cold cereals** can be a rich source of complex carbohydrates and fiber. They are also low in fat, but many are high in sodium. Whole-grain cereals are particularly nutritious, but, again, study the label for sodium levels. Those who eat cereal frequently should check labels for the fat and sodium contained in a single serving. DASH recommends selecting cereals with fewer than three grams of fat and at least three grams of fiber per serving. It is important to restrict dietary sodium in persons with hypertension or heart failure; cereals with low sodium or no sodium, such as old-fashioned rolled oats, can be selected.

- Most **crackers and cookies** have considerable amounts of fat. Some are advertised as being low in fat or fat free, but this claim may be deceptive and confuse the person trying to lose weight, since the calories lost by removing fat may be replaced or even increased by adding sugar to enhance flavor and texture. Salt is also usually added. Again, read labels, and be alert to items containing butter, coconut or palm oil, or shortening, all of which are high in fat and calories. Also, be aware that some crackers contain a high amount of sodium; however, crackers with reduced sodium are available.

- **Breads** contain little or no fat, but some contain significant amounts of sodium (salt is added to bread because it speeds up the leavening process). Choose breads that contain low or no sodium. Or consider baking your own, and reduce the salt content.

- **Frozen meals and dinners** may be high in calories, especially if they contain foods that are breaded or fried. DASH recommends frozen dinners containing 400 to 600 calories, 10 to 15 grams of fat, and less than 800 milligrams of sodium per serving. Healthy Choice, Lean Cuisine, and Smart Ones are considered wise choices.

- **Frozen desserts,** such as sherbets, low-fat ice cream, and frozen low-fat yogurt, are low in calories and healthy. Healthy Choice offers a variety of low-fat ice creams that are especially tasty and are recommended by DASH.

Remember that reducing fat, calories, and salt from a recipe does not mean you destroy flavor. The DASH eating plan suggests adding herbs (parsley, thyme, basil, sage, rosemary, tarragon, mint, cilantro, and chives), spices, mustard, balsamic or flavored vinegars, nonfat vanilla yogurt, nonfat sour cream, a mixture of Parmesan and mozzarella cheese, and extra fresh or frozen vegetables to your cooking. Fruits also enhance the taste of meals with few additional calories. Adding flavor in this way can make a significant difference in improving the taste of food.

The "S" Culprits

In short, if you want to improve your nutrition and health, make note of the foods and behavioral factors that are especially linked to obesity, type 2 diabetes, stroke, heart disease, kidney disease, hardening of the arteries, and many common cancers—*and then make changes in your lifestyle to avoid or significantly reduce these foods and behaviors.* Think of them as the twelve "S" culprits:

1. sugar
2. sweets and other foods high in carbohydrates
3. sodas and other drinks sweetened with fructose
4. saturated fats
5. snacks that are calorie-dense
6. salt
7. serving sizes that are too large
8. second helpings
9. spirits and other alcoholic beverages
10. sedentary lifestyle
11. smoking
12. sleep deficiency

. . . .

If at first you fail to lose weight, keep trying. With the proper eating and drinking plan, adequate exercise, motivation, persistence, and perseverance, you can succeed!

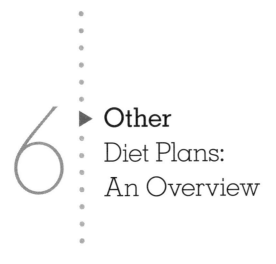

6

▶ Other Diet Plans: An Overview

▶ It is beyond the scope of this book to discuss in detail the many weight-loss diets aggressively marketed throughout this country. However, some of the more popular plans deserve mention. That's the topic of this chapter.

Weight-loss diets encompass a remarkably wide range of approaches, and controversy continues regarding which is preferable and whether any of them should be recommended. All of the weight-loss programs summarized here recommend moderate exercise in addition to the various diets.

Atkins Diet

The Atkins diet consists of a high-protein, high-fat, and low-carbohydrate diet (60 percent of calories from fat, about 10 percent from carbohydrate, and 25 to 30 percent from protein).[1] Metabolizing or burning up body fat on this low-carbohydrate diet produces chemicals called ketones that suppress appetite and sometimes cause nausea, fatigue, and a sweet breath odor. Dr. Atkins believed firmly that foods that markedly elevate blood sugar ("high glycemic foods"), and thereby stimulate insulin release from the pancreas, play the major role in weight gain and should be limited. He believed these foods increased hunger and failed to suppress the desire to eat.

Approximately fifty million Americans have tried a high-fat, low-carbohydrate diet such as the Atkins diet. Furthermore, a number of Atkins grocery items have been sold in a variety of food outlets, and the T.G.I. Friday's chain of restaurants worked with the Atkins organization to produce low-carbohydrate menu items. The Atkins diet apparently causes a greater weight loss for the first six months than a low-fat/high-carbohydrate diet such as the Ornish diet; however, after one year, weight loss was not significantly different from a calorie-controlled low-fat diet. In one study, about 40 percent did not stay on the Atkins diet.

The Atkins diet should not be followed by persons with impaired kidney or liver function, since it may aggravate kidney failure or liver disease. Furthermore, as Dr. Atkins indicated, the diet should not be used during pregnancy or when mothers are nursing. Although in the short run the diet may *decrease* blood cholesterol levels in some, cholesterol levels may become significantly elevated. Its effects on heart health, cancer risk, and diabetes are unclear. This diet limits consumption of fruits and certain vegetables, rich sources of antioxidants, which are important in preventing and combating a variety of diseases.

The original Atkins diet did not make a distinction between "good" and "bad" fat, and the diet permitted consumption of both. However, more recently, because of years of scientific criticism, representatives of Atkins have altered the original diet program that permitted consumption of unlimited fat and red meat. They now recommend smaller portions of meat and limiting saturated fat to 20 percent of total calories. Saturated fat is mainly present in meat, cheese, butter, and shortening; the remaining dietary fat should come mainly from vegetable oil and fish. Although this revision is healthier than the original Atkins diet, the plan is still considerably higher in protein and fat than is recommended by most medical professionals and registered dietitians. The evidence that a high-fat diet causes hardening of the arteries and may play a role in the cause of colon cancer is compelling, and there is evidence suggesting that excess cholesterol in the diet may increase the risk of Alzheimer's disease. Prolonged consumption of high-fat foods can damage arteries in the heart and brain and cause heart disease and stroke. Furthermore, prolonged consumption of a high-protein diet may increase loss of calcium from bone, which is undesirable, especially in those with decreased bone calcium or osteoporosis. It is noteworthy that low-carbohydrate diets also afford very little fiber, which may result in constipation and increase risk of some diseases of the colon, such as an irritable bowel, diverticulitis, and even cancer. Furthermore, vitamin supplements may be required to prevent vitamin deficiencies in people who follow the Atkins diet or other low-carbohydrate diets.

An emphasis on the importance of eating "low-carb" diets is unfortunate and misleading; it is not the answer for long-term weight loss. Scientific studies show that most people can lose weight on a "high-carb" diet, as long as they mainly consume good (unrefined) carbohydrates (e.g., whole-grain foods, fruits, vegetables, legumes, breads, cereals, brown rice, whole wheat pastas). These carbohydrates are highly nutritious and have a relatively low glycemic index—that is, they do not increase glucose (blood sugar) very much. They can be consumed in normal amounts without causing weight gain. Sugars and foods containing sugar have a low to moderate glycemic index, whereas starches (e.g., white bread, white rice, potatoes) are low in nutrients but have a high glycemic index, and their consumption should be limited. (See the section on the South Beach Diet starting on page 104 for a more-detailed discussion of the glycemic index.)

Ornish and Pritikin Diets

The Ornish diet, developed by Dr. Dean Ornish, prescribes a very low-fat, high-carbohydrate diet (10 to 15 percent of calories from fat, more than 65 percent from carbohydrate, and 10 to 20 percent from protein).[2] This diet avoids sugars and refined carbohydrates (e.g., sugar, white flour, white rice, and white bread) but advocates carbohydrates in their whole or complex forms (e.g., beans, brown rice, whole grains, fresh fruits and vegetables, nuts, unrefined whole-wheat bread), which also are rich in antioxidants and fiber. Certain types of fiber help lower cholesterol levels, and a high-fiber diet may lessen the chances of developing colon cancer. Some may find it difficult to adhere to a diet so low in fat for an extended period of time. A low-fat diet is not recommended for children under two years of age, since at a young age the nervous system requires adequate fat for normal development. There are no long-term concerns with a very low-fat diet.

The Pritikin weight-loss program, developed by Robert Pritikin and his father, Nathan, is in many ways similar to the Ornish diet program. It emphasizes limiting fat, choosing the right carbohydrate-rich foods that are high in fiber (e.g., vegetables, fruits, and whole grains), choosing low-fat dairy products, and eating frequently (to avoid hunger).

Recently, a multi-medical center study of three hundred obese men and women ages eighteen to sixty-five, without any serious illness such as diabetes or abnormal blood fats, demonstrated that weight loss of about 7 percent could be achieved by consuming *either* a low-carbohydrate *or* a low-fat diet for two years, if combined with adequate physical activity (mostly walking) and adherence to the diets.[3] It is noteworthy that HDL (good cholesterol) increased and diastolic blood pressure decreased significantly more in those on the low-carbohydrate diet than in those on the low-fat diet. No other significant differences were reported. It was concluded that a low-carbohydrate diet is a viable option for treating obese adults. However, 32 percent of participants on the low-fat diet and 42 percent of those on the low-carbohydrate diet did not remain on these diets for two years. This suggests that remaining on these diets for a prolonged period can be difficult for some.

More palatable diets, such as the DASH eating plan, are more acceptable for prolonged adherence. Especially important for losing weight with any eating plan is to reduce calories by limiting portion size, especially of calorie-dense foods, and to decrease saturated fats and sugar in foods and drinks.

South Beach Diet

Dr. Arthur Agatston's South Beach Diet is neither a low-fat nor a low-carbohydrate diet. He correctly emphasizes balanced meals that contain good fats (monounsaturated and polyunsaturated fats such as olive, canola, and peanut oil, low-fat dairy products, and nuts) and good carbohydrates (such as whole-wheat bread, whole-wheat pasta, and most cereals). He urges avoiding sugar and avoiding or limiting products made with white flour (such as white bread and pasta), potatoes, and white rice. Usual amounts of lean beef, pork, veal, lamb, chicken, turkey, fish, shellfish, vegetables, fruits, and desserts are permitted. Snacks between meals are also recommended. The South Beach Diet seems reasonably balanced and more palatable than the Atkins or Ornish diets.

Dr. Agatston also emphasizes limiting foods with a high glycemic index. As mentioned above, the glycemic index (GI) measures how much the blood glucose increases in response to various foods. Starchy foods have the highest GIs since the carbohydrate they contain is composed of 100 percent glucose. However, table sugar, termed sucrose, is composed of 50 percent glucose and 50 percent fructose and therefore causes a smaller increase in GI than starchy foods, since fructose does not increase blood glucose. In general, processed starches such as white rice, white bread, dry cereal, and snack chips have a high GI, whereas legumes and unprocessed grains have a moderate GI, and nonstarchy vegetables and fruits have a low GI. When carbohydrate foods are tested separately, they trigger different glucose responses, but when they are eaten in a meal, the differences are blunted. The use of the GI for meal planning is controversial. Some small studies have shown beneficial results on blood glucose control, but other larger, longer-term studies have not found the same beneficial effects. Long-term studies comparing high- or low-GI diets for weight loss report identical weight losses. The American Diabetes Association states that there is not sufficient evidence of the benefits of relying on the glycemic index to recommend its use.

The South Beach Diet, unlike the Atkins Diet, avoids both "bad carbs" and "bad fats." Persons starting this diet are required for the first two weeks to avoid foods with a high glycemic index (e.g., bread, rice, potatoes, pastas, baked goods, fruit, candy, cookies, ice cream, and sugar); protein and healthy fats are permitted. According to Dr. Agatston, avoiding foods with a high glycemic index can cause eight to thirteen pounds of weight loss and correct the way the body reacts to foods that increase weight. However, we are unaware of any research to support his claims. After two weeks some of these "bad carbs" are permitted again, and the diet is continued until the target weight is achieved. A more liberal diet is continued thereafter to maintain the weight loss. Except for the elimination or reduction of "bad carbs" and "bad fats," the South Beach Diet recommendations for maintaining target weight are quite similar to what most Americans usually eat. That makes the diet more palatable and acceptable than other weight-loss diets.

The concept that the body can be reprogrammed in two weeks to resolve insulin resistance caused by excess consumption of "bad carbs" is theoretical and not scientifically proven. Other factors influence blood sugar levels—for example, age, weight, physical activity, and the combination of foods consumed at a meal.

Nutrisystem

Nutrisystem is another weight-loss program based on the glycemic index of various foods. Prepackaged entrees and snacks contain "good" carbs (those with a low glycemic index), optimal amounts of protein and fiber, and are low in fat. Customers can supplement these items with some fruits, vegetables, and dairy products. Healthy portion and calorie control is maintained, and the meals are said to prevent pronounced elevations of blood glucose and insulin and also to reduce cravings for foods between meals. The idea is to give the customer limited responsibility for planning meals, grocery shopping, and cooking.

Although it is likely that persons strictly adhering to the Nutrisystem program will lose weight, the long-term success of the program has not been established. Most people may be unable to adhere to the program for long because Americans frequently dine at restaurants and at other people's homes. And individuals who have to cook for others in their family may find it tempting to stray off of the Nutrisystem plan and eat some of the food they're preparing.

Weight Watchers

Weight Watchers is a group program that focuses on losing excess weight by decreasing calories, usually based on a point system assigned to various foods. Members participating in the program are given a certain number of points based on their height, current weight, age, and activity level. Physical activity earns extra points. Participants who attend meetings pay about forty dollars monthly; online participation costs about eighteen dollars per month. A lifetime member may attend meetings free of charge if a healthy weight is maintained.

As an alternative to the point system, participants are taught healthy eating, which includes limiting certain foods rather than limiting the quantity of foods.

Jenny Craig

The Jenny Craig weight-loss program supplies prepackaged meals that are meant to be supplemented with fruits, vegetables, and low-fat dairy products. Meals contain 50 to 60 percent of calories from carbohydrates, 20 to 25 percent from protein, and 20 to 25 percent from fat. An increase in physical activity is also encouraged. Participants who are trying to lose weight are contacted to help them implement the program. The goal is not only to promote weight loss but also to teach people to prepare healthy meals and to serve appropriate portions on their own so that they can maintain their weight loss. The program is relatively expensive and does not limit salt consumption. In addition, it can be difficult to learn how to cook healthy meals similar in caloric content to the small, prepared meals supplied by the program.

The Zone and Sugar Busters Diets

Dr. Barry Sears' Zone Diet claims that maintaining certain ratios of dietary carbohydrate to protein and fat will result in an improved balance of insulin and certain other hormones, leading to weight loss. However, no evidence validates these claims. Those following this diet will lose weight because it is low in calories and emphasizes vegetables and fruits.

Mr. H. Leighton Steward proposes that cutting sugar (the Sugar Busters eating plan) is important for losing weight. But, as has been pointed out by many nutrition experts, lumping foods such as potatoes, corn, and carrots with refined sugar in cakes, candies, and sodas goes too far. The diet also encourages eating saturated fat and decreasing vegetable consumption, which in the long run is unhealthy.

. . . .

There are no long-term studies on the benefits or effectiveness in maintaining weight loss caused by any of the popular weight-loss diets. The bottom line is that calories count! To lose weight, you must cut back on the amount of calories consumed and become more physically active. Maintaining a desired weight requires an ongoing effort to avoid both excess calorie consumption and a sedentary lifestyle. Most people cannot continue to follow these diets; they regain and sometimes go on to gain more than the weight they have lost.

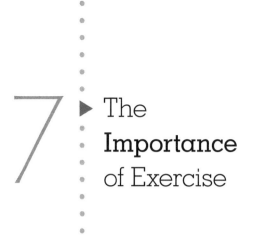

7 ▶ The Importance of Exercise

▶ As you probably know very well, there's another crucial piece of the health-and-well-being puzzle besides diet: physical activity. Exercise is essential for health and physical fitness. Unfortunately, Americans recently have become passive spectators rather than active participants in physical activities, exercise, and sports.

About 40 percent of adults do not engage in any leisure-time physical activity. Furthermore, adults, children, and teenagers have become obsessed with television, computers, computer games, cell phones, and other electronic devices. These are major contributors to the erosion of physical activity in our society. Eating high-calorie foods and drinking sugary sodas or other beverages while watching TV, and consuming lots of buttered popcorn, nachos, candy, and other high-calorie foods and sodas at the movies or sporting events compounds the health consequences of physical inactivity and contributes significantly to weight gain and obesity. The tens of thousands of spectators at a football game need exercise, but only the twenty-two players on the field are getting any.

Bottom line: Physical fitness is essential for good health and longevity. It also provides an overall sense of well-being, even during periods of rest between exercise sessions.

Get Children Moving

About 25 percent of children in America spend four or more hours per day watching television, and many spend seven hours a day in front of a TV or computer screen. Surprisingly, some children age three or younger watch TV between two and three hours daily. During these years, the brain of a child is rapidly undergoing nerve growth and developing connections; although it's not conclusively proven, recent evidence suggests that excess exposure to TV at this young age may influence brain development and result in difficulty concentrating (attention deficit) during school years and later. It is recommended that children two years old or younger do not watch TV. For older children, the American Academy of Pediatrics recommends limiting TV and video viewing to no more than two hours daily. The reality, however, is often quite different, as the following statistics demonstrate:[1]

- A study of ten-year-old American girls revealed a direct correlation between hours spent watching TV and excess body fat.

- A survey in one city revealed that 60 percent of children had a TV in their room, and that they were three times more likely to be overweight than those without TVs. Other statistics indicate that 70 percent of young people have a TV in their room, and 50 percent have a video game player.

- A 2010 report indicated that almost two-thirds of young people ages eight to eighteen said the TV is usually left on during meals, and half of them said the TV was left on "most of the time" in their homes.

- Young people spend over fifty-three hours per week watching TV and using video games and computers.

The increasing time spent in front of computers further erodes participation in physical activities and reduces physical fitness. More statistics:

- Only 27 percent of high-school students engage in moderate physical activity for at least thirty minutes daily for five or more days each week.
- Only 22 percent of adults exercise for at least thirty minutes during most days.
- Up to 80 percent of Americans do not exercise regularly, and 40 percent do not exercise at all.

Physical inactivity exerts a particularly strong influence on the development of obesity in children. Of great concern is that three-fourths of children who are overweight or obese at ages nine to thirteen will remain so when adults. It appears that inadequate physical activity, especially among individuals with lower levels of education and income, is a contributor to obesity. Surprisingly, recent studies have found that many people living in the suburbs are more obese than those living in cities. Apparently, suburbanites constantly use cars for transportation, since stores and shopping centers are often miles away from their homes. Furthermore, because sidewalks are often unavailable in the suburbs, suburbanites walk much less frequently than city dwellers.

There has been an unfortunate trend for public schools in the United States to decrease or eliminate PE (physical education) in the belief that more time for academic instruction is preferable. This is a very serious mistake that must be reversed. Besides PE during school hours, after-school programs are extremely important for the health and welfare of our children. Most children and teenagers who get into trouble by smoking, using drugs and alcohol, committing crimes, and becoming involved in fights or serious gang activity do so between 3:00 and 6:00 PM. Responsible supervision of young people during this critical time period is crucial, and playing sports or engaging in other physical activities is an ideal way both to keep kids occupied and to promote their health. Physical exercise is important not only for physical health but also for mental health since it can reduce emotional tension and provide a sense of well-being. Unfortunately, some school administrators may curtail unsupervised exercise activities on school property to minimize the chances of injury and subsequent lawsuits against the school for "inadequate supervision."

Parents, schools, and the government should demand regular physical exercise periods for all students. It is especially valuable if parents can participate with their children in extracurricular and community physical activities and sporting events. This will help children practice and enjoy regular exercise.

Schools often emphasize team sports and the importance of winning. As a consequence, some children and teenagers with limited athletic ability or who aren't naturally competitive but who would enjoy participating in sports or other fitness activities are left idle on the sidelines with little or no exercise and with poor self-esteem and a sense of inferiority. Such inactivity must not be permitted; every child and teenager should be involved regularly in an exercise program. Although competitive sports are very popular, not all physical activity must be done in a competitive environment; other sorts of physical activity may be preferred by some children. Encouragement can do wonders for children and teenagers; none should be left behind.

What Type of Exercise Should You Do?

Sedentary persons ("couch potatoes") are more likely than those who are physically active to be overweight or obese and eventually to develop hypertension, heart attacks, strokes, diabetes, and elevated harmful fats in the blood. The good news for those who don't yet have an exercise habit is that exercise doesn't have to be performed at intense levels to help prevent these conditions. Moderate-intensity training is just as effective as, if not better than, high-intensity exercise in providing many beneficial effects.

What type of exercise should you do? The best answer is anything you enjoy. That way you will be more likely to stick to it. Make sure your activity of choice includes an aerobic element. Aerobic exercise is dynamic exercise that increases oxygen intake and increases activity of the heart, lungs, and muscles.

The benefits of regularly performing moderate aerobic exercise are many:

- Proper weight is more easily achieved and maintained.

- Muscle mass, strength, and agility are increased and preserved, reducing the chance of falls and injuries.

- The risks of osteoporosis and diabetes are diminished. Weight-bearing activities, e.g., walking, running, jogging, weightlifting, etc., are important in protecting against osteoporosis. (Swimming, although an excellent muscle exercise, is not weight-bearing and is not protective against osteoporosis. It is noteworthy that the weightlessness occurring in space flights causes astronauts to lose considerable amounts of calcium in their urine.)

- Elevated blood pressure may be reduced.

- Damage to the coronary arteries of the heart may be prevented, heart function improved, and the chance of a heart attack decreased in both men and women.

- Levels of the "good" blood cholesterol (HDL, i.e., high-density lipoprotein), which protects against hardening of the arteries, may be increased, whereas levels of the "bad" cholesterol (LDL, i.e., low-density lipoprotein) and triglycerides (blood fats) usually decrease.

- Emotional tension, anxiety, anger, and depression may be significantly alleviated; the chance of heart attack and sudden death caused by excessive emotional or physical stress may be reduced.

- The occurrence of colon and breast cancer may be decreased.

- Inflammation and pain may be reduced in the joints of patients with some types of arthritis.

- Mental decline in the elderly may be delayed.

Researchers have shown that exercise benefits the heart by improving the ability of the heart arteries to dilate in response to a substance (nitric oxide) released from the lining of the arteries. This dilation occurs even in the presence of atherosclerosis (hardening of the arteries). Furthermore, it has been reported that "regular moderate exercise not only increases muscle utilization of energy, but also enhances formation of new nerve cells in areas of the brain that support memory."[2] Finally, researchers at Harvard recently reported that increased physical fitness in children improved their academic performance.

One of my patients was under considerable stress as an executive in his company. At the end of each workday, he would return home, walk into the woods nearby, and scream for prolonged periods. This was his way of releasing anxiety and frustration. He had no time for exercise or relaxation, he said, and he hardly ever took a lunch break. When I discovered that he had been a track star in college, I urged him to find time to jog regularly. He did so, and he told me that jogging had an enormous beneficial effect on his life and on his relationships with his family and associates.

Exercise intensity and duration for adults should be increased gradually and then performed for thirty or more minutes, at least five or preferably all days of the week. For children, sixty minutes of moderate physical activity most (preferably all) days of the week is recommended. Individuals older than forty years or anyone with any indication of heart or vascular disease should consult a physician before embarking on an exercise program. A variety of stress tests can provide valuable information about the coronary arteries and function of your heart and the degree to which you can safely exercise. Furthermore, your physician probably will check your blood levels of sugar and cholesterol, and may determine levels of homocysteine and C-reactive protein, chemicals that may be involved in hardening of the arteries. Any elevations of these chemicals may require medication with drugs, such as the statins, which can lower elevated levels of the bad cholesterol and C-reactive protein; folic acid can lower homocysteine.

Walking and jogging are particularly popular types of exercise that can be performed alone, with a few friends, or in large groups. To determine how far you have walked, jogged, or run, simply multiply your stride (measured in feet from toe to toe or heel to heel) times the number of strides accumulated on a pedometer attached to your belt during the exercise. In fact, a pedometer can be very helpful in tracking physical activity for everyone. Most adults should take ten thousand steps daily to maintain adequate physical activity.

Bicycling, basketball, soccer, tennis, paddle tennis, swimming, squash, volleyball, cross-country skiing, skating, roller-blading, golf (especially if walking rather than using a cart), group aerobic exercise, and dancing are all excellent exercises that improve cardiovascular fitness and muscle strength. Even regularly performed light-intensity exercise, such as tai chi, may reduce blood pressure modestly. To keep most physically fit, exercises should be periodically varied so that all the major muscles will be strengthened.

Exercise machines (such as the treadmill, rowing machine, stationary bicycle, stair climber, and the vast array of dynamic muscle-building machines) are excellent and very convenient ways to work out; the opportunity to watch television, listen to music, or even read while using these machines can enhance the enjoyment of exercise. Most of these moderate-intensity exercises pose little chance of injury, especially if a few minutes of muscle stretching—a warm-up period—precede the exercise. Stretching after exercise is also beneficial in preventing muscle soreness and stiffness.

If you walk or jog on a road, a word of caution regarding the use of an iPod or similar device: The possibility of being hit by a car is increased if your hearing is impaired. Especially if you're listening to an iPod, jogging or walking is safer if done against traffic so that you can see and avoid oncoming vehicles.

Whatever sort of exercise you decide to pursue, bear in mind that it is especially important to choose enjoyable activities; if you find them boring, you won't continue them for long.

Exercise and Blood Pressure

Although exercise will briefly increase systolic blood pressure, systolic and diastolic pressures may be lower for as long as several hours after the activity ends. (See Chapter 4 for a definition of "systolic" and "diastolic" blood pressure.) In hypertensive subjects, regular, moderate aerobic exercise can reduce systolic and diastolic blood pressure by about 10 mm and 8 mm Hg (mercury), respectively. No evidence suggests that regular, moderate-intensity exercise increases the risk of stroke or heart attack in individuals with mild hypertension who have no heart disease or previous history of vascular disease of the brain. However, exercise may have to be limited for those with heart disease or other disabling conditions. If hypertension is severe, it should be controlled with antihypertensive medication before embarking on an exercise program.

Lifting or "pressing" very heavy weights will build skeletal muscles; however, the straining required with this sort of exercise, known as isometrics (requiring extreme muscle contraction), may need to be avoided, especially if you have hypertension. Strenuous isometrics can elevate both systolic and diastolic pressures, with systolic pressure sometimes reaching 300 mm Hg or higher. Severe elevations of blood pressure could be especially hazardous for anyone taking aspirin or anticoagulants. Repetitive light weightlifting or exercises requiring intermittent contraction and relaxation of muscles, if not strenuous, are permissible. Moderate isometric exercise is desirable because it can maintain a muscular body that burns more calories than a fat body and can help prevent overweight and obesity. Physical fitness can also increase agility and prevent falls.

Most antihypertensive (blood pressure–lowering) medications do not interfere with the ability to exercise. However, some drugs that partially block the response of the heart to exercise, such as beta blockers, will limit the pumping action of the heart and slow the pulse. Consequently, these drugs may reduce a person's capacity for strenuous physical activity.

Calorie Burning

Exercising with moderate intensity for thirty minutes will burn approximately 150 calories in a person of average weight. If it works better for your schedule on any given day to perform two fifteen-minute or three ten-minute periods of exercise, the benefit derived and the total calories burned will be similar. Men burn 10 to 20 percent more calories than women during exercise, probably because of men's larger muscle mass. The number of calories burned also depends on a person's weight, the type and intensity of exercise, and the time spent exercising. Table 12 on the next page shows the approximate number of calories a person would expend in thirty minutes performing various physical activities, broken down by the person's weight (because a heavier person expends more calories than a lighter person performing the same amount of exercise).

Table 12. Exercise Calorie Expenditures, Sorted by 30-Minute Activity and Body Weight

Activity	Weight (in lbs.)													
	120	130	140	150	160	170	180	190	200	220	240	260	280	300
Aerobic dancing (low impact)	138	149	161	172	184	195	207	218	230	253	276	299	322	345
Aerobics step training, 4" step (beginner)	174	189	203	218	232	247	261	276	290	319	348	377	406	435
Aerobics, slide training (basic)	180	195	210	225	240	255	270	285	300	330	360	390	420	450
Badminton	180	195	210	225	240	255	270	285	300	330	360	390	420	450
Basketball (game)	264	286	308	330	352	374	396	418	440	484	528	572	616	660
Basketball (leisurely, nongame)	156	169	182	195	208	221	234	247	260	286	312	338	364	390
Bicycling, 10 mph (6 min/mi)	150	162	175	188	200	213	225	237	250	275	300	325	350	375
Bicycling, 13 mph (4.6 min/mi)	240	260	280	300	320	340	360	380	400	440	480	520	560	600
Billiards	54	58	63	68	72	76	81	85	90	99	108	117	126	135
Bowling	66	72	77	82	88	94	99	105	110	121	132	143	154	165
Canoeing, 2.5 mph	84	91	98	105	112	119	126	133	140	154	168	182	196	210
Canoeing, 4.0 mph	162	175	189	202	216	230	243	257	270	297	324	351	378	405
Croquet	72	78	84	90	96	102	108	114	120	132	144	156	168	180
Cross country snow skiing, intense	396	429	462	495	528	561	594	627	660	726	792	858	924	990
Cross country snow skiing, leisurely	186	202	217	232	248	263	279	294	310	341	372	403	434	465

Table 12. Exercise Calorie Expenditures, Sorted by 30-Minute Activity and Body Weight (cont'd.)

Activity	Weight (in lbs.)													
	120	130	140	150	160	170	180	190	200	220	240	260	280	300
Cross country snow skiing, moderate	264	286	308	330	352	374	396	418	440	484	528	572	616	660
Dancing (fast)	120	130	140	150	160	170	180	190	200	220	240	260	280	300
Dancing (slow)	66	72	77	82	88	94	99	105	110	121	132	143	154	165
Gardening, moderate	108	117	126	135	144	153	162	171	180	198	216	234	252	270
Golfing (walking, without cart)	120	130	140	150	160	170	180	190	200	220	240	260	280	300
Golfing (with a cart)	84	91	98	105	112	119	126	133	140	154	168	182	196	210
Handball	276	299	322	345	368	391	414	437	460	506	552	598	644	690
Hiking/back-packing with a 10 lb load	216	234	252	270	288	306	324	342	360	396	432	468	504	540
Hiking/back-packing with a 20 lb load	240	260	280	300	320	340	360	380	400	440	480	520	560	600
Hiking/back-packing with a 30 lb load	282	306	329	352	376	399	423	446	470	517	564	611	658	705
Hiking, no load	186	202	217	232	248	263	279	294	310	341	372	403	434	465
Housework	108	117	126	135	144	153	162	171	180	198	216	234	252	270
Ironing	60	65	70	75	80	85	90	95	100	110	120	130	140	150
Jogging, 5 mph (12 min/mi)	222	240	259	278	296	315	333	352	370	407	444	481	518	555
Jogging, 6 mph (10 min/mi)	276	299	322	345	368	391	414	437	460	506	552	598	644	690
Mopping	102	111	119	128	136	144	153	162	170	187	204	221	238	255
Mowing	162	175	189	202	216	230	243	257	270	297	324	351	378	405

(cont'd.)

Table 12. Exercise Calorie Expenditures, Sorted by 30-Minute Activity and Body Weight (cont'd.)

Activity	Weight (in lbs.)												
	120	130	140	150	160	170	180	190	200	220	240	260	280	300
Ping Pong	108	117	126	135	144	153	162	171	180	198	216	234	252	270
Raking	90	98	105	112	120	128	135	142	150	165	180	195	210	225
Racquetball	246	266	287	308	328	349	369	389	410	451	492	533	574	615
Rowing (leisurely)	90	98	105	112	120	128	135	142	150	165	180	195	210	225
Rowing machine	216	234	252	270	288	306	324	342	360	396	432	468	504	540
Running, 8 mph (7.5 min/mi)	366	396	427	458	488	518	549	579	610	671	732	793	854	915
Running, 9 mph (6.7 min/mi)	396	429	462	495	528	561	594	627	660	726	792	858	924	990
Running, 10 mph (6 min/mi)	420	455	490	525	560	595	630	665	700	770	840	910	980	1050
Scrubbing the floor	168	182	196	210	224	238	252	266	280	308	336	364	392	420
Scuba diving	228	247	266	285	304	323	342	361	380	418	456	494	532	570
Shopping for groceries	72	78	84	90	96	102	108	114	120	132	144	156	168	180
Skipping rope	342	370	399	428	456	484	513	541	570	627	684	741	798	855
Snow shoveling	234	253	273	292	312	332	351	371	390	429	468	507	546	585
Snow skiing, downhill	156	169	182	195	208	221	234	247	260	286	312	338	364	390
Soccer	234	253	273	292	312	332	351	371	390	429	468	507	546	585
Squash	246	266	287	308	328	349	369	389	410	451	492	533	574	615
Stair climber machine	192	208	224	240	256	272	288	304	320	352	384	416	448	480
Stair climbing	168	182	196	210	224	238	252	266	280	308	336	364	392	420
Swimming (25 yds/min)	144	156	168	180	192	204	216	228	240	264	288	312	336	360

Table 12. Exercise Calorie Expenditures, Sorted by 30-Minute Activity and Body Weight (cont'd.)

Activity	Weight (in lbs.)													
	120	130	140	150	160	170	180	190	200	220	240	260	280	300
Swimming (50 yds/min)	270	292	315	338	360	382	405	428	450	495	540	585	630	675
Tennis	192	208	224	240	256	272	288	304	320	352	384	416	448	480
Tennis (doubles)	132	143	154	165	176	187	198	209	220	242	264	286	308	330
Trimming hedges	126	136	147	158	168	178	189	199	210	231	252	273	294	315
Vacuuming	90	98	105	112	120	128	135	142	150	165	180	195	210	225
Volleyball (game)	144	156	168	180	192	204	216	228	240	264	288	312	336	360
Volleyball (leisurely)	84	91	98	105	112	119	126	133	140	154	168	182	196	210
Walking, 2 mph (30 min/mi)	72	78	84	90	96	102	108	114	120	132	144	156	168	180
Walking, 3 mph (20 min/mi)	96	104	112	120	128	136	144	152	160	176	192	208	224	240
Walking 4 mph (15 min/mi)	120	130	140	150	160	170	180	190	200	220	240	260	280	300
Washing the car	90	98	105	112	120	128	135	142	150	165	180	195	210	225
Waterskiing	192	208	224	240	256	272	288	304	320	352	384	416	448	480
Waxing the car	120	130	140	150	160	170	180	190	200	220	240	260	280	300
Weeding	120	130	140	150	160	170	180	190	200	220	240	260	280	300
Window cleaning	90	98	105	112	120	128	135	142	150	165	180	195	210	225

(Source: Adapted from http://sandy.utah.gov/fileadmin/downloads/administration/slim_down_sandy/2009/Exercise_Calorie_Expenditures.pdf; http://www.acefitness.org/acefit/healthy_living_tools_content.aspx?id=9; http://www.mayoclinic.com/health/exercise/SM00109.)

To lose weight, it is essential to reduce daily calorie consumption in addition to exercising. Regular physical activity is essential for a healthy heart and vascular system, but the number of calories burned during exercise is relatively small and incapable of significantly reducing weight. Without caloric restriction, physical activity will not effectively reduce excess weight.

A good measure of fitness is your heart rate and the length of time you can continue on a treadmill at different degrees of exercise. A person's maximum heart rate (pulse) during exercise decreases with age. To calculate your heart rate in beats per minute, immediately after exercise count the pulse rate at your wrist for six seconds, and multiply the number by ten. With moderate exercise, this number in the normal, healthy individual should be roughly equivalent to 220 minus your age (the formula for maximum rate), multiplied by 70 percent (the recommended percent of the maximum rate that should be attained during moderate exercise):

$$(220 - \text{age in years}) \times 0.7 = \text{maximum target heart rate}$$

Report any abnormalities of heart response to exercise to a physician.

. . . .

Obviously, the adage "no pain, no gain" does not apply to exercise. Regularly performed, moderately intense, nonpainful exercise can be both enjoyable and beneficial to health. Strenuous exercise is not required or recommended to lose weight and stay fit. So, if there are no medical reasons to avoid or limit physical activity, start exercising regularly and discover the many ways to enjoy it!

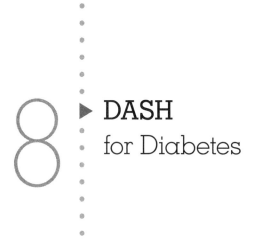

8 ▶ DASH
for Diabetes

▶ Just as eating healthfully is important for the general public, it also is very important for persons with diabetes. Besides its benefits for controlling blood pressure and reducing weight, the DASH diet can be a very effective eating plan for managing type 2 diabetes. The American Diabetes Association recommends an eating pattern that includes carbohydrate from fruits, vegetables, whole grains, legumes, and low-fat or skim milk—as does the DASH food plan.

If you have diabetes, you want an eating plan that can help you control your blood glucose, cholesterol, blood pressure, and weight. To keep your blood glucose as normal as possible, you need to balance the foods you eat (especially the carbohydrates), your physical activities, and the insulin your body makes or gets by injection. Blood-glucose monitoring provides the information you need to help with this balancing act. Physical activity also helps improve your health and your blood glucose levels. Review Chapter 7 for ideas about how to be more active every day. *(Note: If you've been diagnosed with diabetes, it is always essential that you consult your physician regarding nutrition therapy changes, and that you obtain the guidance of a registered dietitian.)*

The Role of Insulin

Foods supply you with the energy needed for all daily activities. That energy is measured in units called "kilocalories"—usually called just "calories." All calories come from carbohydrate, protein, and fat, and food is made up of some proportion of each of these "macronutrients," as they're termed. The hormone insulin, made and released by the beta cells of the pancreas, is needed for these nutrients to be used correctly. Incidentally, calories can also come from alcohol, but alcohol, when consumed in moderation, does not affect blood glucose levels and does not require insulin for the body to use.

Carbohydrate in foods is primarily absorbed through the intestinal wall as glucose, which then goes to the liver. The glucose can leave the liver and be carried by the bloodstream to the cells of the body, where it is used as an immediate source of energy. It can also be stored in the liver or muscles in the form of glycogen. Glycogen can later be converted back to glucose and used for energy. Glucose that is not needed as an immediate energy source or stored as glycogen is changed by the liver to fat and stored in fat cells for future energy needs. Insulin is needed for this whole process to take place.

Three types of carbohydrates are found in food: starches, sugars, and fiber. Starches are found in breads, cereals, pastas, legumes, and starchy vegetables. Sugars are either added to foods or "naturally occurring," which are found in fruits, vegetables, and milk. Fiber gives structure to foods and cannot be digested by the body. It is the balance between sugars and starches eaten and available insulin that primarily determines what blood glucose levels will be after eating meals or snacks. Many research studies have shown that the total amount of carbohydrate eaten is more important than the type, and this is the basis for carbohydrate counting discussed later in the chapter.

Animal and vegetable proteins from food are broken down in the intestine into amino acids, which go to the liver. Some amino acids are used to make new bodily tissue for growth and repair. Some are stored in the liver as glycogen and can be used when needed for energy. Excess amino acids can also be changed to fat and stored. This whole process also requires insulin.

Fats in foods are a combination of three fatty acids and are called triglycerides. After fat is absorbed through the intestinal wall it also goes to the liver and then to the fat cells to be stored and used when needed as a source of energy. Insulin allows triglycerides to enter the fat cells for storage. If not enough insulin is available, or if a person has developed resistance to insulin, levels of triglycerides and cholesterol will often be elevated. There are three kinds of fatty acids: saturated, monounsaturated, and polyunsaturated. Saturated (and *trans*) fatty acids raise blood cholesterol and cause insulin resistance and so should be avoided when possible.

Insulin, therefore, is crucial to the body's use of carbohydrate, protein, and fat. Although food carbohydrates affect blood glucose levels after eating, it is important for people with diabetes to also be careful of the total amounts of protein and fat they eat. The best advice is to eat healthy foods in appropriate portion sizes.

If you have type 1 diabetes, your pancreas no longer can make enough insulin and, therefore, you must take insulin by injection or by an insulin pump to control your blood-glucose levels. If, by contrast, you have the much more common type 2 diabetes, your pancreas is still producing insulin, but your body has become resistant to its actions—a condition called "insulin resistance." This may be mainly due to the extra body fat that most people with type 2 diabetes gain with age. As long as your body can make the increased amounts of insulin needed to overcome the insulin resistance, your blood glucose will remain normal; however, if your pancreas cannot make enough insulin, diabetes develops. Because over time your pancreas produces less and less insulin, most individuals with type

2 diabetes usually need to take more than one medicine to control their blood glucose and may need to take insulin as well. But regardless of your medications, paying attention to proper eating, losing excess weight, and being more physically active continue to be important.

How DASH Can Help

It is helpful for most people with diabetes to eat meals (and snacks, if desired) at regular times every day. Your daily carbohydrate intake should be about the same from day to day. If you use insulin or other glucose-lowering medications, you should avoid skipping meals and overly restricting carbohydrates. Doing either can cause your blood-glucose levels to drop too low.

People with diabetes find that "carbohydrate counting" helps them plan their meals and control their blood-glucose levels. The DASH food plan meshes well with carbohydrate counting. One carbohydrate serving is the amount of food that contains 15 grams of carbohydrate. A recommended starting point is for men to eat four to five carbohydrate servings at a meal and women three to four. If you choose to snack, one carbohydrate serving is usually appropriate. You may find you need more or fewer carbohydrate servings for your meals. The number of carbohydrate servings as well as the amount of calories, protein, and fat you require are determined by many factors, such as your weight, activity level, and medical conditions (e.g., pregnancy, recovery from an illness or surgery, or serious infection).

Table 13 lists the food groups and the number of daily servings recommended for the DASH eating plan and the serving sizes recommended for carbohydrate counting.

The next step is to develop a plan of eating that meets your needs. A registered dietitian can help you do this. The sample menu outlined in Table 14 on page 129 is an example of combining the DASH plan and carbohydrate counting.

Table 13. Food Groups, Recommended Number of Daily Servings, and Serving Sizes for Carbohydrate Counting

Food Groups and Servings per Day	Serving Sizes
Carbohydrate Foods	**Examples of a 1 Carbohydrate Serving**
Grains, grain products, starchy foods, starchy vegetables (such as potatoes, corn, winter squash, peas), legumes (beans and lentils) *7–8 each day*	1 oz of a bread product, such as a slice of bread ½ small bagel, English muffin, or pita bread ½ small hamburger bun or hot dog bun 1 6 in tortilla 4–6 crackers ½ C* cooked cereal, grain, or starchy vegetable ⅓ C cooked rice or pasta ¾ C dry cereal ½ C cooked beans, lentils, peas, or corn 1 small potato (3 oz) ½ C sweet potato or yam 1 C soup ¾ oz pretzels, tortilla chips, or snack crackers
Fruits *4–5 each day*	1 small fresh fruit (4 oz) ½ C fresh, frozen, or canned fruit ¼ C dried fruit ½ C fruit juice 1 C melon ¾ C berries 1¼ C strawberries
Vegetables, nonstarchy (average serving sizes contain small amounts of carbohydrate and do not need to be counted as a carbohydrate serving) *4–5 each day*	1 C raw vegetables ½ C cooked vegetables ½ C tomato or vegetable juice
Low-fat or nonfat dairy foods *2–3 each day*	1 C nonfat or low-fat milk (8 fluid oz or ½ pt) ⅔ C (6 oz) nonfat or low-fat yogurt (plain or flavored with an artificial sweetener)
Sweets *5 per week*	⅓ C sherbet 3 pieces hard candy ½ C light ice cream Small piece (2 oz) angel food cake 2 small cookies (2¼ in across)

(cont'd.)

Table 13. Food Groups, Recommended Number of Daily Servings, and Serving Sizes for Carbohydrate Counting (cont'd.)

Food Groups and Servings per Day	Serving Sizes
Meat and Meat Substitutes	**Serving Sizes**
Meat, Poultry, Fish *6 oz or less each day (3 oz is an average serving size of meat, poultry, or fish and equals the size of a deck of cards)*	1 oz cooked lean mean, poultry, or fish ¼ C fat-free or low-fat cottage cheese ¼ C tuna 1 slice low-fat cheese 1 egg ⅓ C tofu
Nuts and Seeds *4–5 servings per week*	1½ oz or ⅓ C nuts ½ oz or 2 Tbsp seeds 1 Tbsp peanut butter or other nut spread
Fats and Oils *2–3 each day*	1 tsp soft margarine 1 Tbsp low-fat mayonnaise 1 Tbsp salad dressing or 2 Tbsp light salad dressing 1 tsp oil (olive, canola, corn, safflower, flax-seed, or other)

* C = cup

This menu contains approximately 2,000 calories. If you require fewer calories, cut out one serving of a food from each meal or cut the snacks. The menu also contains less than 2,000 mg sodium (assuming you don't shower everything with copious amounts of table salt). This is less than the 2,300 mg sodium intake recommended for the general public but more than the 1,500 mg found to be most beneficial in the trial of reducing sodium on the DASH eating plan. But it is also much less than the 3,500 to 5,000 mg sodium that most Americans typically consume each day. Cutting back on sodium is a big step in the right direction for overall health. Even getting down to 2,000 to 3,000 mg sodium daily, combined with eating more fruits and vegetables (which are high in potassium) and low-fat or nonfat dairy foods, will have a beneficial effect on your blood pressure based on the research done on the DASH eating plan.

Fortunately, eating more fresh (versus highly processed) vegetables, fruit, and dairy foods automatically lowers sodium intake. Very

Table 14. Carbohydrate Counting and DASH (Sample Menu, Carbohydrate Servings, and Food Groups)

Breakfast:
1 small banana (1 carbohydrate serving)
¾ C* Cheerios (1 carbohydrate serving)
1 C nonfat or skim milk (1 carbohydrate serving)
1 slice whole wheat toast (1 carbohydrate serving) with 1 Tbsp peanut butter (1 nut serving)
Totals: 4 carbohydrate (1 fruit, 2 grains, 1 dairy) servings and 1 nut serving

Lunch:
1 pita bread (2 carbohydrate servings)
¾ C chicken salad for sandwich (2 oz meat and 1 fat serving)
Raw vegetables: 3–4 carrot sticks, 3–4 celery sticks, 2 lettuce leaves (2 nonstarchy vegetable servings)
1 C nonfat milk (1 carbohydrate serving)
1 small apple (1 carbohydrate serving)
Totals: 4 carbohydrate (2 grains, 1 dairy, 1 fruit) servings, 2 nonstarchy vegetables, 2 ounces of meat, and 1 fat serving

Dinner:
1 medium-size serving of lean roast beef (3 oz of meat)
½ large baked potato (2 carbohydrate servings)
1 Tbsp sour cream or 1 tsp soft margarine (1 fat serving)
½ C steamed broccoli (1 vegetable serving)
1 spinach salad: ½ C raw spinach, 2 cherry tomatoes, ½ C sliced cucumber (1 vegetable serving)
1 Tbsp olive oil and vinegar salad dressing (1 fat serving)
1 small whole-wheat dinner roll (1 carbohydrate serving)
1 C melon balls (1 carbohydrate serving)
Totals: 4 carbohydrate (2 starchy vegetables, 1 grain, 1 fruit), 2 nonstarchy vegetables, 3 oz of meat, 2 fat servings

Snacks (morning, afternoon, evening, or added to meals):
¼ C dried apricots (1 carbohydrate serving)
1 C low-fat yogurt (1 carbohydrate serving)
1¼ C strawberries (1 carbohydrate serving)
3 C plain popcorn (1 carbohydrate serving)
2 Tbsp mixed nuts (1 fat serving)
Totals: 4 carbohydrate (2 fruit, 1 dairy, 1 grain) servings, 1 fat serving

Totals for the day:
16 carbohydrate servings (8 grains and starchy vegetable, 5 fruit, 3 dairy)
4 nonstarchy vegetable servings
2 meat servings (5 oz)
2 nut servings
4 fat servings

* C = cup

little sodium is found in fresh foods. Processed foods contribute the most—up to 80 percent of the sodium in most diets, whereas only 20 percent comes from the salt shaker and unprocessed food.

Useful Tips for Selecting Portion Sizes Based on Carbohydrates

The following are some general tips for selecting portion sizes:

- For many foods from the grain list (bread, rolls, buns, bagels, muffins), 1 ounce equals 1 serving. Because of their large size, some foods have more carbohydrate (and calories) than you might think. For example, a large bagel may weigh 4 ounces and equal 4 carbohydrate choices.

- 1 small fresh fruit; ¼ cup dried fruit; ½ cup fresh, frozen, or canned fruit; or ½ cup fruit juice are 1 carbohydrate servings. Portion sizes for canned fruit are for the fruit and a small amount of juice (1 to 2 tablespoons).

- Different types of milk and milk products are included on the "Dairy Food" lists. However, two types of dairy products are found in other lists. Cheeses are included on the "Meat and Meat Substitutes" list because they contain protein and fat and very little carbohydrate. Cream and other dairy fats are on the "Fats" list.

- Many sugar-free, fat-free, or reduced-fat foods are made with ingredients that contain carbohydrate. Such foods often have the same amount of carbohydrate as the regular foods they are replacing. Be aware—they may have more sodium as well, so check the food label.

- Although sweets may be substituted for other carbohydrate foods, they do not have as many vitamins, minerals, and fiber as other starches, fruits, or milk foods. Some will also have additional amounts of fat. Avoid regular (nondiet) soft drinks with high amounts of carbohydrate.

- Fresh and frozen vegetables have much less salt than canned vegetables and are preferred. When you do eat canned vegetables, drain and rinse them several times to remove some of the salt.

- Meat and meat substitutes (cheese, cottage cheese, eggs) are divided, based on the amount of fat they contain, into lean, medium-fat, and high-fat meats. Whenever possible, choose lean meats. Plant-based proteins are also on this list. Many plant-based proteins also contain carbohydrate, so be sure to read the food label.

- Fats are divided into three groups, based on the main type of fat they contain: unsaturated fats (monounsaturated fats and polyunsaturated fats), saturated fats, and trans fats. A fat serving contains 5 grams of fat and 45 calories. Limit serving sizes and choose unsaturated fats for good nutrition.

- A "free" food is any food or drink choice that has fewer than 20 calories and 5 grams or fewer of carbohydrate per serving. Examples are typical serving sizes for nonstarchy vegetables.

- Many foods are combinations, such as casseroles. In general, 1 cup (8 ounces) of a casserole-type dish (tuna noodles, lasagna, spaghetti with meatballs, chili with beans, macaroni and cheese) is counted as 2 carbohydrate and 2 meat choices.

Note: Whenever possible, select high fiber and/or whole-grain foods in place of processed carbohydrate foods with added sodium, fat, and/or sugar. These foods provide vitamins, minerals, and other healthy substances. Examples are whole-wheat breads, brown rice, and high-fiber cereals.

Useful Tips for Understanding and Using Food Label Information

The following list provides tips for reading food labels and using the information to plan your food selections:

- Check the serving size on the label. Is this about the serving size you plan to eat? All of the information on the label is based on this serving size. The number of servings contained in the package is indicated after the serving size.

- Look at the grams of total carbohydrate in one serving size, and determine the number of carbohydrate choices in that serving size. Remember that 1 carbohydrate choice—such as 1 grain, fruit, or milk serving—equals 15 grams of carbohydrate. Ignore the grams of sugar, as they are included in the total grams of carbohydrate.

- Foods with more than 3 grams of fiber per serving are good sources of fiber.

- Look at the grams of fat in one serving size. Remember that 1 fat choice is based on a serving size containing 5 grams of fat. Look for foods that are low in saturated fat, trans fat, and cholesterol. Select foods with:

  - 3 or fewer grams of fat for every 15 grams of carbohydrate
  - 3 or fewer grams of fat for every 7 to 8 grams of protein (for 1 ounce of meat or meat substitute)
  - ⅓ or less of the total fat as saturated fat

- Look for servings of food that have fewer than 480 milligrams of sodium, and combination foods or meals that have fewer than 800 milligrams.

· · · · · · · · · ·

In summary, use the DASH food plan to help take care of your diabetes, high blood pressure, cholesterol and lipid abnormalities, and excess weight. We and other authorities[1] believe it is the most healthful and acceptable eating plan.

- Eat a wide variety of foods every day, including fruits, vegetables, whole grains, beans, and low-fat dairy foods. Choose high-fiber foods and fresh fruits and vegetables.

- Choose foods with less added fat, sugar, and salt. When you do eat sweets, count them as carbohydrate choices.

- Remember, 1 carbohydrate choice equals 15 grams of carbohydrate.

- Eat meals and snacks at regular times every day, especially if you are taking glucose-lowering medications for diabetes. Keep the amount of carbohydrate in your meals consistent.

- Aim for thirty minutes or more of physical activity nearly every day.

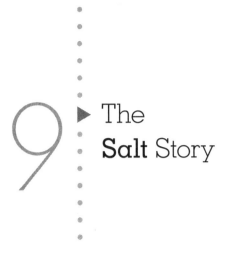

9 ▶ The Salt Story

▶ "If too much salt is used for food, the pulse hardens." Such was an admonition that appeared in the Chinese Yellow Emperor's classic of internal medicine about 2,500 BC. Even that long ago, salt (i.e., sodium chloride, or NaCl) was used as a condiment for seasoning, and it was found to be a valuable preservative. The word "salt" derives from the Latin *sal*. The words "salary" and "salutary" are also derivatives of *sal*.

A Brief History of Salt

Because salt was so valuable, it was used as a form of barter and payment. The Greeks bought slaves with salt, and salt was considered by some to be worth twice its weight in gold. The salt tax in France contributed to the causes of the French Revolution. Gandhi led a protest in India against a salt tax in 1930. In medieval England,

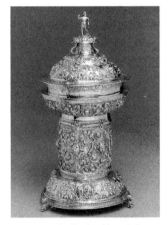

FIGURE 17. Ancient salt container (Image copyright © The Metropolitan Museum of Art. Image source: Art Resource, NY)

to be seated at a dining table "above the salt"—that is, near the elegant salt container (see Figure 17)—was considered a mark of rank and favor. The terms "not worth his salt" and "that should be taken with a grain of salt" are well-known expressions that further suggest the historical importance of salt.

Human beings have existed for 3.5 million years, and for 99.8 percent of that time they were herbivorous—that is, they subsisted on leaves and plants, which were rich in potassium and contained very little sodium (unless they lived by a saltwater sea). It is estimated that prehistoric humans consumed about 700 milligrams (0.7 grams) of sodium and 11,000 milligrams (11 grams) of potassium per day, whereas modern humans consume about 4,000 milligrams (4 grams) of sodium and only 2,500 milligrams (2.5 grams) of potassium (see Table 15).

Table 15. Comparative Consumption of Sodium Versus Potassium

	Prehistoric Humans	Modern Humans
Sodium	0.7 g/day	4.0 g/d
Potassium	11.0 g/d	2.5 g/d
Table Salt (NaCl)	1.75 g/d	10.0 g/d

Subsequently, we have become carnivorous (i.e., flesh eating) and omnivorous (i.e., consuming animals and vegetables). Salt hunger was experienced by some herbivores because of salt deficiency, and treks were made to salt licks in order to augment salt intake. Primitive tribes consumed very small amounts of salt; they apparently did not like salt when first exposed to it. Salt is an acquired taste, and now in acculturated societies the practice of adding salt is ubiquitous; practically all processed foods contain salt, which is composed of 40 percent sodium and 60 percent chloride. Cultural factors have played a central role in creating a salt appetite—an appetite that can be altered upward or downward by increasing or decreasing salt intake. Humans require remarkably little salt unless there is excessive loss in certain disease states or with excess perspiration during strenuous exercise or severe heat exposure. Humans need less than 1 gram (i.e., 1,000 milligrams) of salt per day, yet Americans consume an average of 10 to 12 grams daily.

Salt Intake and Blood Pressure

There is compelling evidence that as salt intake increases, blood pressure rises. Salt is important in causing high blood pressure in perhaps 50 to 60 percent of persons with hypertension. For example, adequate salt reduction or increased salt elimination caused by diuretics ("water pills") can significantly lower blood pressure in some human hypertensives, and there are epidemiological studies indicating a strong correlation between the amount of salt consumption and hypertension. Finally, in certain experimental animal models (especially in rats and even in apes), there is unequivocal evidence that excess salt consumption causes hypertension. (References to human hypertension, as I use the term here, refer to primary hypertension, also termed essential hypertension. The precise cause of essential hypertension, which accounts for 90 percent of all cases of hypertension, remains unknown.)

Particularly informative was a 1948 report by Dr. Walter Kempner, who placed a group of hypertensive patients on what was called a rice diet, which contained practically no salt. Seventy-one percent of the patients had a marked decrease in blood pressure. Those who remained on the rice diet had a significant reduction of their blood pressure, and many who would have died because of their hypertension survived.[1]

Figure 18 reveals a close correlation between salt intake and blood pressure in populations from several geographical areas where there are significant differences in dietary salt consumption.

Dr. Louis Dahl noted that hypertension was uncommon in persons consuming less than 4 or 5 grams of salt per day.

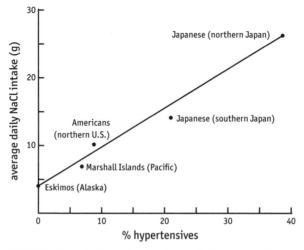

FIGURE 18. Percent of hypertensives in populations consuming various amounts of dietary salt.[2]

Even in the same geographic regions, sometimes a strong correlation exists between the amount of salt consumed and the development of hypertension. Examples of this are found in Japan, Iran, Africa, South America, and the Polynesian and Solomon Islands, where segments of the population consuming diets high in salt have significantly higher blood pressures and hypertension than those on low-salt diets. Moreover, of the six societies of Melanesians studied in the Solomon Islands, systolic and diastolic blood pressures were highest in the society ingesting large quantities of salt, i.e., 8.7 to 13.3 grams daily (similar to acculturated societies) from seawater used in cooking.[3]

The Yanomamo Indians, who inhabit the tropical equatorial rainforest in parts of Brazil and Venezuela, do not use salt in their diet. Some excrete as little as 2 milligrams of sodium per twenty-four hours. Their blood pressures increased from the first to second decade of their lives, but unlike in civilized populations their blood pressures did not increase during subsequent years. These natives also have elevated hormone levels (i.e., plasma renin and urinary aldosterone) as occurs in civilized persons placed on a low-sodium diet. However, that they are seldom obese and remain highly physically active are also factors that could contribute to their low blood pressures, which ranged from 88 to 122 mm Hg systolic and 40 to 72 mm Hg diastolic.

It is worth emphasizing that any time the dietary habits of a group change and there is an increase in the consumption of salt, there is a corresponding increase in the incidence of hypertension in a significant segment of the population: those who are salt sensitive. A good example of the effect of acculturation is seen in nomadic warriors from Kenya who entered the army; when exposed to the higher-salt diets in the army, their systolic blood pressure rose significantly after only two years. However, it is difficult to assess the significance of salt in causing hypertension in Western societies, where a high salt intake is common to almost all and begins in childhood. To perform a meaningful correlation between salt intake and hypertension in an acculturated society would require that one separate those persons who are salt-sensitive from those who are relatively salt-resistant. (Note that almost all people respond to an increased salt intake with some rise in blood pressure; however, some respond more than others and are designated salt-sensitive.) Despite the difficulty in separating these two groups, evidence has been presented by an international cooperative study (Intersalt Study) on fifty-two centers, each with two hundred men and women, from thirty-two countries to establish a significant correlation between the intake of salt and the level of blood pressure even in these acculturated societies. Twenty-four-hour urine-excretion studies revealed a highly significant correlation between sodium excretion and systolic and diastolic blood pressures.[4] A decreased urinary potassium was also significantly correlated with higher systolic blood pressure.

There is no question that genetic susceptibility plays a crucial role in development of hypertension in experimental animals and in humans. Children of hypertensive parents are at very high risk for developing hypertension. However, environmental factors, particularly salt consumption and obesity, also can play major roles in increasing blood pressure. Other environmental factors that can influence blood pressure include sedentary lifestyle, excess alcohol and tobacco consumption, stress, and consumption of certain drugs. Although it was previously thought that the sodium ion alone was responsible for elevating blood pressure, it now appears that the combination of sodium and chloride is essential for the development of hypertension. It is also noteworthy that potassium consumption can lower blood pressure. A deficiency of calcium or magnesium may also contribute to an elevated blood pressure; however, the interaction of sodium, potassium, calcium, and magnesium in blood pressure regulation remains unclear.

The Physiology of Hypertension: Some Theories

Why is there a higher incidence and greater virulence of hypertension in African Americans than in whites? Why do black Americans excrete a sodium load more slowly than whites and consume less potassium than whites? No one knows for certain, but there are some possible explanations. It appears that the kidneys of blacks retain more salt. One theory is that natural selection favored those African captives who could conserve salt in the horrific conditions of the slave ships. As a result, they survived. Those who could not usually perished, probably from salt-depletive diseases, such as diarrhea, vomiting, and fevers. The survivors then passed on to subsequent generations of African Americans an unfortunate capacity to retain excess salt and thus a tendency to develop hypertension. There is as of yet no certainty why blood flow through the kidneys of blacks is diminished because of increased resistance in the arteries of the kidneys. Furthermore, some blacks may consume less potassium than whites, which may explain in part why African Americans have more severe hypertension: Potassium appears to oppose the accumulation of sodium in the body and can dilate arteries and decrease blood pressure.

Although poorly understood, evidence suggests that in some humans and experimental animals hypertension may result from activation of the sympathetic nervous system and retention of salt by the kidneys caused by increased insulin in the blood. There is a large overlap in the occurrence of obesity, diabetes, and hypertension; 80 to 90 percent of people with type 2 diabetes and 60 percent of essential hypertensives are overweight. There is, however, no compelling evidence to implicate insulin in the cause of hypertension.

About one-third of the U.S. adult population suffers from hypertension, and it is estimated that up to 60 percent of these are salt-sensitive. Salt sensitivity is also common in individuals who are obese, who have diabetes, and who are older than sixty-five. In the normotensive population (people with normal blood pressure), about 32 percent of blacks and 30 percent of whites are salt-sensitive, whereas in hypertensives 73 percent of blacks and 55 percent of whites are salt-sensitive.

The only way to discover your sensitivity to salt is to see whether going from a low-salt to a high-salt diet increases your blood pressure or vice versa. There is no precise agreement on the definition of salt sensitivity in humans; however, the most widely applied definition (that recommended by the National Institutes of Health) states that, after seven days on a low-salt diet (containing about 0.6 grams of NaCl) followed by seven days on a high-salt diet (containing about 13.8 grams of NaCl), a 10 percent or greater rise in mean arterial blood pressure indicates salt sensitivity. The mechanism for salt sensitivity has not been determined; however, neurogenic, hormonal, and altered vascular (blood vessel) membrane permeability to sodium have been implicated.

Clinical studies have identified 55 to 65 percent of people with essential hypertension as "nonmodulating" salt-sensitive hypertensives. The kidneys of these persons seem unable to increase (modulate) their blood flow adequately to excrete excess dietary sodium. It is interesting that 85 percent of nonmodulators have a familial history of hypertension, whereas only 25 to 30 percent of modulators (those whose kidneys can modulate—i.e., adequately eliminate—ingested salt) have a family history of hypertension.

The hallmark of many types of experimental hypertension in animals is a reduced ability of the kidneys to excrete adequate amounts of sodium at normal levels of blood pressure. Studies have focused on the mechanism of salt-induced hypertension in salt-sensitive rats developed by Dr. Louis Dahl. These rats provide valuable experimental models of salt sensitivity that is genetically determined and seems quite similar to nonmodulating human essential hypertension.

Several important facts have emerged from these studies. First, when challenged with excessive dietary salt (8 percent NaCl), the kidneys are unable to eliminate the salt load adequately. This retention of salt and water results initially in expanded blood volume, which increases the pumping action of the heart. Moderately severe hypertension is then sustained by constriction of arteries. On the other hand, if salt-sensitive rats ingest a diet of only 1 percent salt for four to nine months, they gradually develop mild hypertension because of arterial constriction, without any increase of blood volume or pumping action of the heart. This latter model of hypertension more closely parallels human hypertension wherein blood volume usually is not expanded and hypertension results from constriction of arteries. Similar mechanisms that cause hypertension in Dahl's salt-sensitive rats may exist in human salt-sensitive hypertension.

Additional investigations indicate that the kidney arteries of salt-sensitive Dahl rats, even before they develop hypertension, are less responsive to agents that dilate the arteries and more responsive to agents that constrict them when compared to Dahl rats that are not salt-sensitive. There is evidence that an inability of the kidney arteries to dilate appropriately in response to excess dietary salt may be due to a genetic defect that results in salt and water retention and thus in development of hypertension in Dahl's salt-sensitive rats.

My colleagues and I have demonstrated a defect in the kidney's handling of sodium that results in salt and water retention, and we have demonstrated that salt-sensitive rats appear to have a deficient generation of a vasodilator (cyclic GMP) when they are placed on a high-salt diet; such a deficiency in the kidney might be responsible for salt and water retention. It has been reported that functional abnormalities of the kidneys (rather than structural changes reported by some) in Dahl's salt-sensitive rats account for salt retention that leads to hypertension. There appears to be no difference between the anatomy of the kidneys of salt-sensitive and salt-resistant rats that might explain the difference in the way their kidneys handle excess dietary salt. It is, therefore, concluded that a functional biochemical issue rather than an anatomical abnormality most likely explains salt retention by the kidneys of salt-sensitive rats.

Some investigators believe that a deficiency of nitric oxide (NO) may play a role in the development of hypertension. When NO is generated from the blood vessels, it stimulates the production of cyclic GMP, which possibly dilates the blood vessels. Therefore, a deficiency of NO generation might possibly explain an apparent deficiency of cyclic GMP.

Although demonstration of a genetic defect in kidneys responsible for sodium retention is central to understanding the cause of salt-induced hypertension, just why retained sodium eventually causes a generalized constriction of arteries and arterioles (very small arteries) that results in hypertension is unclear. One explanation is that the release of a ouabain-like substance (a substance similar to digitalis) into the circulation may cause accumulation of sodium and calcium in arteries, which could result in vasoconstriction and hypertension.

Dietary Recommendations

Because of the magnitude of the problem of salt-induced hypertension and the risk of heart disease and stroke, many experts recommend that a strong effort should be made to limit salt consumption on a national level. Efforts to curtail excess salt consumption in Finland have been very successful, and similar efforts are progressing in the UK, Ireland, Japan, and Portugal. A human's physiological need for salt under normal circumstances is only about 0.58 grams per day; however, in the United States the average man and woman consumes about 10.4 and 7.3 grams of salt per day, respectively. Approximately 90 percent of Americans consume more salt than recommended. A restaurant meal may contain more salt than should be consumed for the entire day. Furthermore, in the past decade, the average sodium content of food has increased about 6 percent. More than 75 percent of the sodium we eat comes from processed food (i.e., food prepared by companies for public consumption) and restaurant meals; about 12 percent comes from natural, unprocessed food, and about 11 percent is added in the household.

Only a cooperative effort of government and industry will curtail salt consumption sufficiently to have a beneficial impact on preventing salt-induced hypertension. It is noteworthy that sodium content labeling on processed food packages increased from 19 percent in 1982 to 60 percent by 1986. Today it is mandatory to list sodium content on all foods that carry a nutrition label; this encompasses 95 percent of all processed and packaged foods. Consumers have a right to know what their food contains. Unfortunately, seventy-two million Americans have hypertension (an increase of over 30 percent since 1994), and, with aging, about 90 percent of Americans will eventually develop hypertension!

Dr. Claude Lenfant, former Director of the National Heart, Lung, and Blood Institute, stated that "damage to arteries begins at fairly low blood pressures—those formerly considered normal."[5] Unfortunately, Americans have steadily increased their sodium consumption in the past twenty years—the result mainly of increased processed-food intake. Higher salt consumption tends to raise blood pressure. Persons with hypertension should read the labels on processed foods to learn the amounts of sodium and chose lower-sodium food items. One also must be aware that the sodium content indicated on the label is for *one* serving—individuals frequently eat more than a single serving. In addition, all should know that the sodium content of fast foods, pizza, and Chinese food is very high.

While everyone needs some salt to function, as mentioned, nearly all Americans consume more than is needed. The U.S. Dietary Guidelines suggest that members of the general population consume no more than 6 grams of salt (2,300 milligrams of sodium) per day. More recently, these guidelines and those written by other authorities recommend that people with hypertension and/or impaired kidney function, people with prehypertension (those with pressures between 120 and 140 mm Hg systolic and/or between 80 and 90 mm Hg diastolic), African Americans, and adults forty years or older limit daily salt consumption to about 3.8 grams (1,500 milligrams of sodium). Furthermore, the American Heart Association recommends that the 2,300 milligrams/day figure is too high and that the goal for all Americans should be no more than 1,500 milligrams of sodium per day.

This prudent recommendation can be achieved by gradually reducing salt consumption by eating more potassium-rich foods (especially vegetables and fruits) and by replacing salt with herbs and other seasonings.

A reduction of sodium intake to 1,500 milligrams (about ½ teaspoon of salt) daily appears both safe and achievable and can decrease the severity of hypertension. The reduction is especially important in the high-risk groups listed above. Restriction of sodium may also reduce the number of people developing hypertension each year by at least 20 percent and decrease the yearly mortality rate from stroke by more than 39 percent and heart attack by more than 30 percent. Reducing dietary sodium increases the effectiveness of certain antihypertensive drugs and may eliminate the need for medication in some hypertensive persons. It has been estimated that reducing the salt consumption of adult Americans by half would save 150,000 lives each year!

Salt, it has been said, "is perhaps the deadliest ingredient in the food supply."[6] The less salt consumed, the greater the protection from the development of hypertension, stroke, heart, kidney, and arterial disease. Salt reduction in children can lower blood pressure, and may prevent hardening of the arteries at a young age. Recent evidence indicates that excess salt consumption may damage the heart and arteries of some, even in the absence of hypertension. Evidence also shows that salt reduction may decrease the risk of enlargement of the heart, heart failure, stroke, stomach cancer, kidney failure, protein in the urine, calcium kidney stones, and osteoporosis.

Limitation of processed and restaurant foods high in sodium, table salt, and salt used for cooking should be accompanied by other healthful lifestyle changes, such as weight reduction, smoking cessation, limited consumption of alcohol, adequate physical activity, and a diet low in saturated fat and cholesterol and high in fiber, fruits, and vegetables—in other words, a diet like the DASH plan. Fresh foods contain very little sodium, and the addition of pepper, spices, herbs, lemon, onion, garlic, vinegar, table wine, horseradish, unsalted mustard, unsalted catsup, and unsalted Worcestershire sauce can flavor food and help break the salt habit. Be aware of the milligrams of sodium in your food, and use more foods labeled "low sodium" or "unsalted." Keeping a record of your sodium consumption can be very helpful in achieving your goal to reduce dietary sodium. Again: Remember that the milligrams of sodium indicated on the label apply to *one* serving. If you consume *two* servings, you will, of course, be consuming twice the amount of sodium.

Some mistakenly think that sea salt (which comes from evaporated seawater) instead of regular salt (which comes from underground deposits) is healthier, since it contains less sodium. But the only real difference between the two is taste; sea salt contains certain minerals (e.g., magnesium and others) that render it more flavorful than table salt. However, it is important to appreciate that the concentration of sodium chloride in sea salt is 98 percent whereas it is 99.9 percent in table salt. Therefore, excessive use of either can cause hypertension and hardening of the arteries, and both should be limited.

The Center for Science in the Public Interest (CSPI), in a report on the sodium content of a hundred popular foods, found that different brands of similar foods often vary widely in sodium content—by as much as 50 to 100 percent or more. It is noteworthy that the public usually cannot recognize these differences in sodium content by taste. Differences reported in some popular foods with high sodium contents include the following:

- A small order of fries at Burger King has almost three times as much sodium as a small order of fries at McDonald's.

- Bumble Bee solid-white albacore tuna has more than twice as much sodium as Crown Prince's product.

- General Mills Honey Nut Cheerios has more than three times as much sodium as Barbara's Bakery Honey Nut O's.

- Safeway Premium Select BBQ Sauce contains about half as much sodium as Kraft BBQ Sauce.

• More sodium is present in small and medium hamburgers at Burger King than at McDonald's.

Likewise, different brands of hot dogs, bacon, crackers, ham, sausage, breads, cheeses, pizzas, frozen foods, salad dressings, spaghetti sauces, salsa, potato and tortilla chips, chicken strips and nuggets, and soups often contain significant differences in salt content. For example, the sodium content of a single slice of pizza may vary from 300 to over 1,000 milligrams. These large variations in the amount of sodium in foods prepared by different companies only emphasize the importance of reading food labels. The sodium in almost all of these foods could be reduced without significantly altering flavor and popularity. The bottom line: Read labels and choose items with less sodium.

Salt substitutes and "lite salt" should not be used without the recommendation of a physician. Many substitutes contain potassium, which may be hazardous to some—particularly those with impaired kidney function or those taking certain antihypertensive drugs that cause potassium retention. The use of salt tablets to counteract salt and water loss, even with excess sweating during physical activity and in hot weather, should be avoided unless recommended by a physician. Individuals who sweat excessively, however, may need to eat salty foods or additional salt.

Marathon running is a relatively safe sport; however, the belief that you should "stay ahead of your thirst" has been replaced by "drink when you are thirsty." Both individuals who are not highly conditioned and trained runners who plan to compete in a marathon should avoid consuming large amounts of water (e.g., more than 13 cups, or 100 ounces) during the race. Studies indicate that slow runners are particularly apt to stop frequently to drink excess water. This can substantially lower sodium concentration in the blood to critical levels, which can cause acute illness with confusion, nausea, and, rarely, seizures, coma, and death. Low salt concentrations in the blood of marathon runners can be prevented if excess water consumption is avoided. Sports drinks may fail to prevent a decrease in salt concentration in the blood because they supply more water than salt. Adequate salt and water consumption during vigorous exercise, military operations, and desert hikes, especially in hot weather, is vital to prevent heat illness and to maintain performance.

For individuals particularly fond of salt, it is comforting to note that limiting salt will in a short time decrease the desire for salty foods. In a brief period, food begins to taste better without excess salt. Use less salt and more herbs and spices when preparing food. Purchase foods low in salt, and ask for foods low in salt when dining out. Remove the salt shaker from the table when in a restaurant, and when at home store it in the cupboard.

The need to reduce salt consumption in the United States should be a top priority since excess salt very significantly contributes to the development of hypertension and its complications of brain, heart, kidney, and blood vessel disease. None of the currently popular diets stress the importance of reducing salt consumption. Only the DASH eating plan emphasizes the importance and benefit of dietary salt reduction, especially in those with hypertension.

Controversy fueled by the Salt Institute (a trade association of salt producers) and a relatively few hypertension experts continues over whether a national policy should be implemented in an attempt to reduce salt consumption in the general population to approximately 4.5 grams or no more than 6 grams per day. The dictum of the medical profession—"first, do no harm" (*primum non nocere*)—must always be paramount in any effort affecting the patient or society. However, there is no evidence that reducing dietary salt to the national goal of 1,500 milligrams of sodium for most people would be harmful, whereas the benefit to our society could be enormous. There is a growing movement led by the Food and Drug Administration, the American Heart Association, the National Institutes of Health, the American Public Health Association, most hypertension experts, and most registered dietitians to recommend moderation of dietary salt (sodium chloride) as one of the four steps to help Americans prevent hypertension; the other steps are maintaining a healthy weight, remaining physically active, and, for those who drink, limiting alcohol consumption to no more than two drinks per day for men and one drink a day for women.

A 2013 report on salt by the Institute of Medicine suggests there is no evidence to indicate that reducing salt consumption to 1,500 milligrams per day reduces deaths from coronary disease or stroke. Unfortunately, in their effort to provide an "evidence"-based report, the IOM document used flawed methodology and did not actually consider all the evidence. They call for a randomized clinical trial, which is not practical or feasible in a free-living population. Observation/population studies, cohort studies, and meta-analyses were not considered.

The IOM report acknowledges that reducing salt in the diet will lower blood pressure and reduce the prevalence of hypertension, but it does not use that as a hard end-point criterion. The report acknowledges the benefits of a sodium intake of 2,300 milligrams per day and suggests that should be the national goal and no lower. Oddly, they cite an Italian study of 250 people with congestive heart failure who were being treated with drugs for their condition. The suggestion was made that these subjects, who were on a low-salt diet, experienced *more* adverse events. This study cannot be generalized to the entire population and be the source for public-health policy.

It remains our opinion—and that of the American Public Health Association, the American Heart Association, and the American Medical Association—that older individuals, African Americans, persons with hypertension and/or diabetes, and those with renal disease would benefit from a sodium intake limited to 1,500 milligrams per day. These persons tend to be salt sensitive and to retain salt more than the general population. It would seem reasonable to especially reduce salt intake in these individuals. The rest of the population would also benefit from the 1,500 mg sodium guideline, which is still much more sodium than the body requires for daily living.

In 1997 Dr. Claude Lenfant, while Director of the National Heart, Lung and Blood Institute (NHLBI), disseminated the following statements:

> "Evidence has accumulated over decades to show a clear causal link between sodium intake and blood pressure."
>
> "Sodium's effect on blood pressure is direct and dose-dependent."
>
> "The evidence comes from basic, epidemiologic, and clinical research, including the NHLBI-supported Trials of Hypertension Prevention and Trials of Nonpharmacologic Interventions in the Elderly."
>
> "The evidence is so strong that it warrants specific public health recommendations about dietary sodium."[7]

Anyone wishing to reduce sodium consumption must read food and beverage labels, select lower-salt foods, and avoid products with a high sodium level. Also, they must limit or not use the salt shaker (see Figure 19).

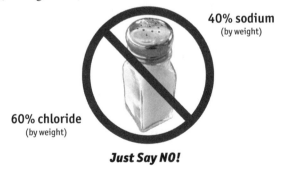

40% sodium
(by weight)

60% chloride
(by weight)

Just Say NO!

FIGURE 19. Table salt (NaCl)

Some common foods and their sodium content are listed in Table 16, which we include as a helpful guide for those wishing to reduce their sodium consumption. Beware of particularly high sources of sodium! These include tomato and V8 juices, cocoa mix, canned soups, canned vegetables, bologna, Italian sausage, smoked meats, spaghetti with meat sauce or meatballs, pot pies, frozen dinners, soy sauce, bacon, frankfurters, ham, tuna in oil, anchovies, sardines, pancake mix, salted potato chips, pretzels, salted popcorn and nuts, English muffins, bread and rolls, pizza, some cereals, waffles, milk, butter, American cheese, bouillon, catsup, dill pickles, sauerkraut, baking powder, and baking soda.

Table 16. Some Common Foods and Their Sodium Levels

FOOD	AMOUNT	SODIUM (mg)
Canned bouillon	1 C*	782
Canned juice, tomato	½ C	438
Canned meat	1 oz	394
Canned soup, chicken noodle	1 C	849
Canned soup, lentil with ham	1 C	1,319
Canned spaghetti and meatballs	1 C	940
Cheeses: Cream Swiss American, processed Low-sodium cheddar or colby	 1 oz 1 oz 1 oz 1 oz	 84 73 405 6
Frankfurter, beef	1 serving	461
Olives, canned	3	120
Pickles, dill	1 spear	384
Pizza, cheese	1 slice	336
Pot pie, beef	1 serving	736
Pot pie, turkey	1 serving	1,390

(cont'd.)

Table 16. Some Common Foods and Their Sodium Levels (cont'd.)

FOOD	AMOUNT	SODIUM (mg)
Salad dressing, thousand island	1 Tbsp	109
Sausage, Italian	1 link	665
Soy sauce	1 Tbsp	1,005
Frozen dinner, fried chicken with mashed potatoes and corn	1 serving	1,500
Frozen dinner, meatloaf with mashed potatoes and carrots	1 serving	1,943

* C = cup
(Source: U.S. Department of Agriculture, Agricultural Research Service. USDA nutrient database for standard reference, release 13, 1999. Nutrient Data Laboratory home page, http://www.nal.usda.gov/fnic/foodcomp.)

· · · · · · · · · ·

Unfortunately, most people seem to pay insufficient attention to limiting dietary salt but are much more concerned with the fats, carbohydrates, and calories they consume. Perhaps their attention can be captured with the following information: Compelling evidence indicates that the increased thirst caused by salty foods frequently results in consumption of high-calorie sugary drinks by adults and children, which plays a significant role in weight gain.

The fact that salt plays such an important role in both the development and severity of hypertension and its complications mandates that greater efforts be made to decrease its use. Increased endeavors are needed to:

1. Inform people with hypertension and the public about the risks of using excess salt.

2. Indicate the salt content of foods consumed in restaurants.

3. Eliminate products containing lots of salt, fats, and sugar from school menus and vending machines, and include water and nonsugary drinks.

4. Curtail the marketing of foods with high salt content.

These efforts may be helpful. However, as the former National High Blood Pressure Education Program and the Center for Science in the Public Interest have repeatedly indicated, the only successful way of decreasing salt consumption is through the reduction of the salt content of processed foods and the introduction of new, palatable foods with much less salt that will be accepted by the public.

▶ Concluding Remarks: Don't Give Up!

Energy and persistence conquer all things.

— Benjamin Franklin

▶ The importance of adhering to a healthy eating plan and engaging in appropriate physical activity cannot be overstated. Doing so is crucial both to turn the tide against the obesity-related complications plaguing our country (hypertension, type 2 diabetes, cholesterol and triglyceride abnormalities in the blood, and many cancers) and to set the example for inspiring healthy habits in our young people. We, along with many other health and nutrition experts, endorse the DASH diet because it is a remarkable multipurpose eating plan that is admirably suited for reducing excess body weight and lowering elevated harmful cholesterol and triglycerides in the blood. Furthermore, with slight modification, DASH can be especially helpful in controlling type 2 diabetes. Embracing this eating plan—combined with obtaining thirty minutes of moderate exercise at least five days per week—can go a long way toward helping you achieve your health goals.

It has been said that motivation is what gets you started, and habit is what keeps you going. But habits usually do not change overnight, so be patient with yourself and with others. Don't give up. If adopting all aspects of a new lifestyle at once seems overwhelming, consider breaking it down into manageable pieces, adding a new piece every week or two. For example, maybe you can start by focusing on boosting fruits and vegetables in your daily diet, in accordance with the DASH plan (see Chapter 4). Once that begins to feel more natural, select another of the major food groups as outlined in DASH, and concentrate on improving your habits in that area. But remember that the DASH plan is meant to be a complete approach to eating, so it's important eventually to incorporate all aspects of it into your dietary habits, to the best of your abilities. Use the same approach with Chapter 5, which is full of pointers for integrating healthy eating into your life. Pick two or three tips, and focus on them until they start to feel natural. Then pick a few more, etc. Work physical activity into your daily habits in the same way. Perhaps start with a fifteen-minute walk three days a week, then build up to thirty minutes five days a week. Habituating yourself gradually to changes can increase the likelihood that they will become permanent.

With the proper motivation one *can* be inspired to change habits. Our experience with the VITAL (Values Initiative Teaching About Lifestyle) program, mentioned in Chapter 1, which teaches healthy eating and appropriate physical activity to very young schoolchildren, has been quite a satisfying reminder of this fact. The program has proven successful in instilling healthy lifestyles and preventing excess weight gain in young children. Its implementation is very easy and fun for all involved.[1] Of course, children's habits are often somewhat easier to influence than adults', but the enthusiastic involvement of parents and teachers in the VITAL program has demonstrated that adults can be motivated to change, too. In fact, a desire to set a good example for their children is usually one of the best motivators for parents when faced with the need to change their own health habits. They recognize that healthy eating and appropriate physical activity are fundamental to maintaining or improving their children's health.

We believe that you, like the participants in the VITAL program, can find the motivation to make changes to benefit your health, and we sincerely hope this book helps you transform that motivation into life-changing habits.

▶ Notes

Chapter 1

1. L. Murtagh and D. S. Ludwig, "State Intervention in Life-Threatening Childhood Obesity," *Journal of the American Medical Association* 306, no. 2 (2011 Jul 13): 206–7.

2. Manu Raj and Krishna Kumar, "Obesity in Children and Adolescents," http://www.ncbi.nlm.nih.gov/pmc/articles/PMC3028965 (accessed 21 August 2013).

3. Assistant Secretary for Planning and Evaluation at the U.S. Department of Health and Human Services, "Childhood Obesity," http://aspe.hhs.gov/health/reports/child_obesity (accessed 21 August 2013).

4. New York City Department of Health and Mental Hygiene, "Obesity in Early Childhood: More than 40 Percent of Head Start Children in NYC Are Overweight or Obese," *NYC Vital Signs* (2006): 496–500.

Chapter 2

1. E. A. Finkelstein et al., "Annual Medical Spending Attributable to Obesity: Payer and Service-Specific Estimates," *Health Affairs (Millwood)* 28, no. 5 (2009): w822–31.

2. Science Daily, "Obesity Accounts for 21 percent of U.S. Healthcare Costs, Study Finds," www.sciencedaily.com/releases/2012/04/120409103247.htm (accessed 21 August 2013).

3. Helen Disney, "Fat Is a Fiscal Issue," http://opinion.publicfinance.co.uk/2007/10/fat-is-a-fiscal-issue (accessed 21 August 2013).

4. Jeffrey Friedman, "A War on Obesity, Not the Obese," *Science* 7, no. 5608 (2003): 856–58.

5. E. C. Koop, "Dietary Guidelines," Chapter 7 in *Sick and Tired? Reclaim Your Inner Terrain,* by Robert O. Young and Shelley Redford Young (Pleasant Grove, UT: Woodland Publishers, 2001).

6. Centers for Disease Control and Prevention, "Obesity and Overweight," http://www.cdc.gov/nchs/fastats/overwt.htm (accessed 21 August 2013).

7. R. H. Unger and P. E. Scherer, "Gluttony, Sloth and the Metabolic Syndrome: A Roadmap to Lipotoxicity," *Trends in Endocrinology and Metabolism* 21 (2010): 345–52.

8. Mary Clare Jalonick, "'Too Fat' for Empire? Military Generals Target School Lunches," http://www.commondreams.org/headline/2010/04/20-4 (accessed 21 August 2013).

9. S. Stabouli, S. Papakatsika, and V. Potsis, "The Role of Obesity, Salt and Exercise on Blood Pressure in Children and Adolescents," *Expert Review of Cardiovascular Therapy* 9, no. 6 (2011): 753–61.

10. M. W. Gillman et al., "Family Dinner and Diet Quality Among Older Children and Adolescents," *Archives of Family Medicine* 9, no. 3 (2000): 235–40.

Chapter 3

1. Jane E. Brody, "In Summer's Heat, Watch What You Drink," http://www.nytimes.com/2010/06/29/health/29brod.html (accessed 21 August 2013).

2. Mayo Clinic, "Soda Consumption Linked to Obesity, Type 2 Diabetes, and Other Health Concerns," http://www.mayoclinic.org/news2010-mchi/5914.html (accessed 21 August 2013).

3. H. K. Choi and G. Curhan, "Soft Drinks, Fructose Consumption, and the Risk of Gout in Men: Prospective Cohort Study," *British Medical Journal* 336 (2008): 309–17.

4. American Society for Metabolic & Bariatric Surgery, "Rationale for the Surgical Treatment of Morbid Obesity," http://asmbs.org/2011/11/rationale-for-surgical-treatment (accessed 21 August 2013); American Association of Clinical Endocrinologists, The Obesity Society, and American Society for Metabolic & Bariatric Surgery, "Medical Guidelines for Clinical Practice for the Perioperative Nutritional, Metabolic, and Nonsurgical Support of the Bariatric Surgery Patient," https://www.aace.com/files/bariatric.pdf (accessed 21 August 2013); Silvio E. Inzucchi, "Diabetes Facts and Guidelines," http://endocrinology.yale.edu/patient/50135_Yale%20National%20F.pdf (accessed 21 August 2013).

5. Denise Grady, "Seeking to Fight Fat, She Lost Her Liver," *The New York Times,* March 4, 2003.

6. J. L. Pilliteri et al., "Use of Dietary Supplements for Weight Loss in the United States: Results of a National Survey," http://www.ncbi

.nlm.nih.gov/pubmed/18239570 (accessed 21 August 2013); H. M. Blanck et al., "Use of Nonprescription Dietary Supplements for Weight Loss Is Common Among Americans," http://www.ncbi.nlm .nih.gov/pubmed/17324663 (accessed 21 August 2013).

Chapter 4

1. L. J. Appel et al., "Effects of Protein, Monounsaturated Fat, and Carbohydrate Intake on Blood Pressure and Serum Lipids: Results of the OmniHeart Randomized Trial," *Journal of the American Medical Association* 294 (2005): 2455–64.

2. Thomas Moore, *The DASH Diet for Hypertension* (New York: The Free Press, 2002), 24.

3. Ibid., 35.

4. J. F. Hollis et al., "Weight Loss During the Intensive Intervention Phase of the Weight-Loss Maintenance Trial," *American Journal of Preventive Medicine* 35, no. 2 (2008): 118–26.

Chapter 5

1. T. Sachiko et al., "Dietary Protein and Weight Reduction," http:// circ.ahajournals.org/content/104/15/1869.full (accessed 21 August 2013).

2. Kurtis Hiatt, "DASH Diet," http://health.usnews.com/best-diet /dash-diet (accessed 21 August 2013).

3. M. P. Longnecker et al., "Risk of Breast Cancer in Relation to Lifetime Alcohol Consumption," *Journal of the National Cancer Institute* 87 (1995): 923–29; Naomi E. Allen et al., "Moderate Alcohol Intake and Cancer Incidence in Women," *Journal of the National Cancer Institute* 101, no. 5 (2009); 296–305.

4. World Life Expectancy, "The Amish Obesity Studies," http://www .worldlifeexpectancy.com/the-amish-obesity-studies (accessed 21 August 2013); G. B. Cuyun Carter et al., "Dietary Intake, Food Processing, and Cooking Methods Among Amish and Non-Amish Adults Living in Ohio Appalachia: Relevance to Nutritional Risk Factors for Cancer," http://www.ncbi.nlm.nih.gov/pubmed/22026912 (accessed 13 August 2013).

5. Erin Beck, "The Effect of Exercise on Appetite Suppression," http:// www.livestrong.com/article/359914-the-effect-of-exercise-on -appetite-suppression (accessed 21 August 2013).

Chapter 6

1. WebMD, "The Atkins Diet," www.webmd.com/diet/atkins-diet-what
   -it-is (accessed 21 August 2013).
2. WebMD, "Review: Eat More, Weigh Less," www.webmd.com/diet
   /ornish-diet-what-it-is (accessed 21 August 2013).
3. G. D. Foster et al., "Weight and Metabolic Outcomes After Two Years
   on a Low-Carbohydrate Versus Low-Fat Diet: A Randomized Trial,"
   Annals of Internal Medicine 153, no. 3 (2010): 147–57.

Chapter 7

1. American Academy of Pediatrics, "Children, Adolescents, and Television—Committee on Public Education," *Pediatrics* 107 (2001):
   423–26.
2. K. I. Erickson et al., "Exercise Training Increases Size of Hippocam-
   pus and Improves Memory," *Proceedings of the National Academy of
   Sciences, USA* 108, no. 7 (2011): 3017–22.

Chapter 8

1. US News, "Diet Plans that Work," http://health.usnews.com/best
   -diet (accessed 21 August 2013); Jacque Wilson, "And the Year's Best
   Overall Diet Is…," http://www.cnn.com/2013/01/08/health/best
   -diets-ranked (accessed 21 August 2013).

Chapter 9

1. The Rice Diet Program, "Rice Diet Founder Dr. Walter Kempner,"
   http://www.ricediet.com/page/view/rice_diet_founder_dr._walter
   _kempner (accessed 21 August 2013).
2. L. Dahl, in *Essential Hypertension: An International Symposium,*
   ed. P. Ciottier and K. D. Bock (New York: Springer-Verlag, 1960), 53.
3. L. B. Page et al., "Antecedents of Cardiovascular Disease in Six Solomon Island Societies," *Circulation* 49 (1974): 1132–46.
4. Stamler et al., "Findings of the International Cooperative Intersalt
   Study," *Hypertension* 17 (suppl I; 1991): I9–15.
5. National Institutes of Health, "NHLBI Issues New High Blood Pressure Clinical Practice Guidelines," www.nih.gov/news/pr/may2003
   /nhlbi-14.htm (accessed 21 August 2013).
6. Center for Science in the Public Interest, "Public Health Group Calls
   for Reducing Sodium in Food Supply by 75 Percent," http://cspinet
   .org/new/201111011.html (accessed 21 August 2013).

7. Personal communication.

Concluding Remarks

1. W. M. Manger et al., "Obesity Prevention in Young Schoolchildren: Results of a Pilot Study," *Journal of School Health* 82, no. 10 (2012): 462–68, http://www.ncbi.nlm.nih.gov/pubmed/22954165 (accessed 25 August 2013).

▶ Resources

For delicious and nutritious recipes consistent with the DASH eating plan, we recommend the following cookbooks. Persons with diabetes should consult with a registered dietitian regarding the appropriateness of consuming various foods.

The Mayo Clinic Williams-Sonoma Cook Book, by John Phillip Carroll (Birmingham, AL: Oxmoor House, 2002). Winner of the Julia Child Cookbook Award, 1999.

The New Mayo Clinic Cookbook: Eating Well for Better Health (2nd ed.), by Mayo Clinic Physicians (Birmingham, AL: Oxmoor House, 2012). Winner of the James Beard Award, 2005.

Fix-It and Enjoy-It Healthy Cookbook: 400 Great Stove-Top and Oven Recipes, by Phyllis Pellman Good (Intercourse, PA: Good Books, 2009).

For those wishing to learn more about the DASH eating plan and to find additional recipes:

The DASH Diet for Hypertension: Lower Your Blood Pressure in 14 Days—Without Drugs, by Drs. Thomas Moore, Laura Svetkey, Pao-Hwa Lin, and Njeri Karanja, with Mark Jenkins (New York: Gallery Books, 2011).

▶ About the Authors

William M. Manger, MD, PhD, FACP, FACC

Dr. Manger received his bachelor of science degree from Yale University in 1944 and his medical degree from Columbia College of Physicians and Surgeons in 1946. Subsequently he spent two years as a medical intern and resident at Presbyterian Hospital in New York City, and he served as a Lieutenant J. G. in the Medical Corps of the Navy for two years. Between 1950 and 1955 he was a Fellow in Medicine at the Mayo Clinic. He obtained a PhD from the University of Minnesota in 1958. He received the Mayo 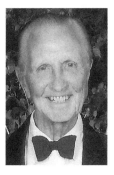 Foundation Alumni Award for Meritorious Research in 1955 for his work on the quantitation of epinephrine and norepinephrine in plasma. Since 1958 he has performed research in areas including: hemorrhagic shock, hypertension, sympatho-adrenal responses, pheochromocytoma, the mechanism of salt-induced hypertension, and the growth of tumor cells.

Dr. Manger has served in the Department of Medicine as Professor of Clinical Medicine at New York University Medical Center since 1983. He is a Lecturer in Medicine (Emeritus) at Columbia Medical School. In 1992 he was designated Distinguished Mayo Foundation Alumnus in recognition of his "exceptional contributions in hypertension for having achieved national and international distinction in research, medical practice, and education and for practicing the high principles which are recognized as exemplary of the Founders of the Mayo Clinic and Mayo Foundation." In 2009 he was awarded the Mayo Clinic Alumni Association Humanitarian Award for his outstanding contributions, dedication, and achievements in improving public health, particularly as a true pioneer in the prevention of childhood obesity, one of the single greatest threats to health in this country. In 2010 he received the PheoPara Alliance Science Award for his research on pheochromocytoma, a treacherous tumor that, if not recognized and removed, can cause hypertension, stroke, heart attack, and death. In 2012 he received the College of Physicians and Surgeons Alumni Association's Gold Medal for excellence in clinical medicine, and the Gold Medal Award of the National Institute of Social Sciences for Distinguished Services to Humanity.

Dr. Manger has a lifelong history of emphasizing the civic message of prevention as the first course of action with chronic illnesses. In 1977 he founded the National Hypertension Association, gradually building up an impressive board of trustees and contributors. Under his leadership the NHA has conducted groundbreaking research on hypertension. Eight years ago, when obesity in children came to the forefront, he and his wife, Lynn, established VITAL (Values Initiative Teaching About Lifestyle) as a humanitarian health measure. The primary purpose of VITAL is to educate children—preschool to third grade—in the prevention of unhealthy lifestyles.

Dr. Manger has written and coauthored five medical books, three books for laypersons, and more than 240 scientific publications.

Throughout his career as a basic researcher and tertiary-care clinician, Dr. Manger has chosen to devote his time, resources, and unbridled energy to improving lives—especially of the underserved and those yet to be served—which are the reasons why the Mayo brothers established the Mayo Clinic.

Other Books Authored or Coauthored by William M. Manger, MD, PhD

Scientific Books
Chemical Quantitation of Epinephrine and Norepinephrine in Plasma (1959)
Hormones and Hypertension (1966)
Pheochromocytoma (1977)
Catecholamines in Normal and Abnormal Cardiac Function (1982)
Clinical and Experimental Pheochromocytoma (1996)

Books for the Layperson
100 Questions and Answers about Hypertension (2001)
Our Greatest Threats: Live Longer, Live Better (2006)
101 Questions and Answers about Hypertension (2011)

— William M. Manger, MD, PhD
Chairman, National Hypertension Association
Professor of Clinical Medicine,
New York University Langone Medical Center
Lecturer in Medicine (Emeritus), Columbia Medical Center

Marion J. Franz, MS, RD, CDE

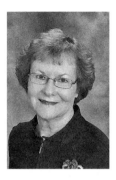

Marion J. Franz is a nutrition/health consultant with Nutrition Concepts by Franz, Inc. For over twenty years she was the Director of Nutrition and Health Professional Education at the International Diabetes Center, Minneapolis. Her Masters Degree in Nutrition is from the University of Minnesota, and she is a Registered Dietitian (RD) and Certified Diabetes Educator (CDE). She has authored over 200 articles, books, booklets, and book chapters on diabetes, nutrition, and exercise, and lectures frequently in the United States and internationally. She is an author of the American Diabetes Association 2006, 2002, 1994, and 1986 nutrition position statements and technical reviews, was a work group member of the American Dietetic Association Evidence-Based Nutrition Practice Guidelines for Type 1 and Type 2 Diabetes 2008, and was editor of the American Association of Diabetes Educators Core Curriculum for Diabetes Education, 4th and 5th editions. She has received numerous awards, including the 2001 American Diabetes Association Charles H. Best Medal for Distinguished Service in the Cause of Diabetes and the 2006 American Dietetic Association Medallion Award.

— Marion J. Franz, MS, RD, CDE
Nutrition/Health Consultant with Nutrition Concepts by Franz, Inc.
Former Director of Nutrition and Health Professional Education
International Diabetes Center, Minneapolis, MN

Jennifer K. Nelson, MS, RD

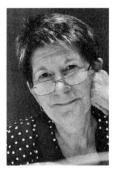

Jennifer K. Nelson is a graduate of the University of Minnesota (BS) and the University of Wisconsin Stout (MS). Her internship was with the U.S. Air Force in Washington, DC, and she was assigned as Chief of Clinical Dietetics at Scott USAF Medical Center in Illinois. She has been in a leadership position at Mayo Clinic for more than fifteen years. She leads clinical nutrition efforts for a staff of more than seventy clinical dietitians and ten dietetic technicians and oversees staffing, strategic and financial planning, and quality improvement. Jennifer is also current Chair of the Minnesota Licensing Board of Dietetics.

In addition to coauthoring the book *The Mayo Clinic Diet,* Jennifer contributes articles and strategic direction to www.MayoClinic.com (Food & Nutrition Center). She was coeditor of the James Beard Foundation award-winning *The New Mayo Clinic Cookbook,* and the Julia Childs award-winning *Mayo Clinic Williams-Sonoma Cookbook* (which also was winner of the 2009 Gourmand World Cookbook Award—Best in Health and Nutrition). She has been a contributing author and reviewer of many Mayo Clinic books, including *Mayo Clinic Healthy Weight for Everybody.* She has also helped develop nutrition materials used by Mayo Health Solutions and their Life Style Coaching program.

— Jennifer K. Nelson, MS, RD
Director, Clinical Nutrition/Dietetics
Associate Professor of Nutrition, Mayo Medical School
Mayo Clinic, Rochester MN

Edward J. Roccella, PhD, MPH

Edward Roccella received his bachelor of science degree from East Tennessee State University. He continued his education at the University of Michigan, where he earned a master of public health and doctor of philosophy degree in health education and health behavior. Wilbur Cohen, former Secretary of Health, Education and Welfare, served as an advisor and a member of Dr. Roccella's dissertation committee. Dr. Roccella began his professional career as Director of Continuing Education at the University 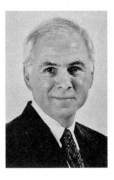 of Pittsburgh Regional Medical Program and as an Instructor in Community Medicine. Subsequently, he became an Assistant Professor at the University of Michigan Medical School and School of Public Health. Since 1978 he has worked at the National Institutes of Health, in Bethesda, Maryland, as Coordinator of the National High Blood Pressure Education Program (NHBPEP). In this position he directed the NHBPEP public, patient, and professional activities, which have been cited to improve the nation's hypertension profile and contributed to the nation's large decline in cardiovascular disease. As NHBPEP Coordinator, he organized forty-five professional, voluntary, and official organizations into one body, which developed national clinical guidelines for prevention and treatment of hypertension, the Joint National Committee reports. He has led United States scientific exchange delegations regarding the prevention and treatment of hypertension to Brazil, Germany, Egypt, and Jordan. Dr. Roccella has authored 107 publications in scientific journals and textbooks dealing with prevention and control of high blood pressure, patient education, public health approaches to improving cardiovascular health, and evaluating large-scale public health programs. He is a past president of the Society for Public Health Education, a former member of the American Public Health Association Governing Council, and serves as a referee for several national and international scientific and medical journals. The Federal Republic of Germany, the Egyptian Ministry of Health, and the Brazilian Ministry of Health have recognized his contributions to hypertension prevention and control.

Dr. Roccella has been awarded the National Institutes of Health Directors Award, the HealthTrac Foundation Prize, the University of Michigan John Romani Prize for lifetime achievement in public health administration, the American Society of Hypertension Presidents Award, the International Society of Hypertension in Blacks Presidential Award, the Society for Public Health Education Distinguished Fellow, and the 2008 Senator Frank Laughtenberg Award. He retired from the National Institutes of Health in 2007 and remains active in the cardiovascular disease prevention and control field and serves on the Medical/Public Health Advisory Boards of four national professional and advocacy organizations.

— Edward J. Roccella, PhD, MPH
Former Coordinator of the National High Blood
Pressure Education Program
Past President of the Society for Public Health Education

▶ Index

Tables and figures are referenced with *t* and *f*, respectively.